Psychodrama, Group Processes and Dreams

'The harmonious combination of psychotherapy theory, dream interpretation, mythology, folklore and metapsychology results in an inspiring work of art.'

Kate Bradshaw Tauvon

Psychodrama, Group Processes and Dreams is the result of years of analytic work with groups and individuals. There are many links between individual and group therapy, group members' personal interactions in and out of the group, and the meanings of dreams. This book introduces us to the dramatic representation of dreams – a new perspective on psychodrama and group therapy – where dramatic action, catharsis and conflict elaboration are of central importance. It is unique in the field of therapeutic practice as it unites Jung's analytical psychology with Moreno's psychodrama. It includes material on:

- The work of Jung and Moreno
- How their theory works in practice
- The constellation of the archetype as transformation.

This unique book enables psychodramatists to incorporate Jungian ideas into their psychodramatic work and gives Jungians a guide to how psychodramatic techniques may help in group therapy. It will also be of great interest to psychotherapists, especially those working in group settings.

Wilma Scategni is a psychiatrist and individual and group psychoanalyst in private practice in Turin, Italy as well as member of the IAAP and IAGP.

Translated by Vincent Marsicano

Psychodrama, Group Processes and Dreams

Archetypal images of individuation

Wilma Scategni
Translated by Vincent Marsicano

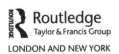
Routledge
Taylor & Francis Group

LONDON AND NEW YORK

Original Italian version – *Psicodramma e terapia di Gruppo: Spazio e tempo dell'anima*, Como: Red edizione (1996)

First published 2002 by Brunner-Routledge
Published 2014 by Routledge
27 Church Road, Hove, East Sussex, BN3 2FA

Simultaneously published in the USA and Canada
by Routledge
711 Third Avenue, New York, NY 10017

Routledge is an imprint of the Taylor & Francis Group, an informa business

Typeset in Times by Keystroke, Jacaranda Lodge, Wolverhampton

British Library Cataloguing in Publication Data
A catalogue record for this book is available from the British Library

Library of Congress Cataloging in Publication Data
Scategni, Wilma, 1946–
   Psychodrama, group processes, and dreams: archetypal images of individuation/Wilma Scategni; translated by Vincent Marsicano.
      p. cm.
   Includes bibliographical references and index.
   1. Psychodrama. 2. Drama–Psychological aspects. 3. individuation (Psychology) in literature. 4. Psychoanalysis and literature.
   I. Title.
   RC489.P7 S286 2002
   616.89′1523–dc21   2001043683

ISBN 978-1-58391-161-7

This book is dedicated to my daughter, Virginia

Contents

Foreword

MARCIA KARP: 'ARTISTIC CREATION LIES WITHIN EACH OF US'

When my daughter was small, she knocked on the door of our bedroom in the early morning. She looked amazed and pleased with herself. She said, querulously, 'Last night I went to sleep and I had all pictures in my head'. It was her first dream. It was her first awareness of her 'head' being able to create something beyond herself, the pictures in a dream. This ability to explore beyond oneself is the strength of the dream. Both Moreno and Jung thought that the goal of the dream is to take the dreamer inside the dream itself. One might ask why it is important to go inside the dream itself. Searching for the meaning of the dream, dreamt beyond the time and space that we know, enriches the time and space we cannot know but wish to. We can make guesses about our lives, but in our dreams we dare to seek answers. By going inside the dream we attempt to make sense of the questions and answers we seek. Sometimes we find their meaning.

When I was 23 years old, Moreno himself directed me in a psychodrama of my dream. I had met him before the dream enactment and was struck by his clarity and wisdom. The night before I began psychodrama training with Moreno and his wife, Zerka, I had to go to the Hamptons in upstate New York to connect with a ride by car to Beacon, New York, where the training began. The Hamptons was a kind of singles cattle market, with young people surveying the goods with an eye to forming relationships. I detested the experience, found it shallow and chose to go to bed early and to meet my car driver (who was enjoying herself on the dance floor as I had tried to do) the next day.

The next day, I took myself and my dream to the new training experience. Before I knew it, Moreno was directing me in the dream. I began by enacting the role I felt just before retiring, a single girl, not happy being perused by the local males. I then performed my role as a potential sleeper, brushing my teeth and getting into bed in preparation for my role as dreamer. I lay on the mattress on the psychodrama stage and was asked by Moreno to first see the dream in my mind as it occurred and then, with the help of the group, to enact it. It involved my family standing on chairs watching me, with a huge cardboard collar around my neck, being eaten by a group of mice with one lead mouse. It was frightening to enact but I had a pleasant feeling of walking around in my own dream. Moreno asked me to lie down on the mattress again and envision the dream as I would like it to be. I got up again and was asked to role reverse with the lead mouse. He had exophthalmic eyes, like Moreno and had his same wisdom. As the eyes bulged, the lead mouse told me, 'You aren't fake. We are here to eat away the cardboard that surrounds you. It isn't yours. You had to put it around yourself in order to get through the Hamptons experience of a meat market for singles.' The director, Moreno, told me to change places with members of my family who were laughing. They assured me that the cardboard person I thought I had to be to exist in the singles night was not the person they knew and loved. They were laughing because I was taken in by the expectations of the singles bar experience.

After the dream was enacted, other group members shared with me similar degrading experiences while trying to catch a partner. By extending the time and space of the night before the dream, I went along a channel of meaning and clarity which helped me make sense of a seemingly meaningless experience. The dream enactment confirmed what I suspected to be true: if I eat away the many layers of expectations, I find the true me still intact.

The next day my colleagues were most intrigued that Moreno had not interpreted the mice and their long tails as phallic symbols. Moreno assured us that the meaning of the symbols lay within the individual dreamer and was to be interpreted by the role reversal of the dreamer. This gave the symbol its meaning, one which was inside the dream.

In this book, we clearly see that artistic creation lies within each of us. What has been created in the past, such as symbols and myths, is there to assist our creation but not to define it. As Scategni sensitively points out, an in-depth exploration of dreams enacted and analysed in the group unfolds in a free associative manner. As it unfolds, the bridge between present time and space gently unfurls, connecting it to the time and space of the soul.

(Marcia Karp is director of the Hoewell International Psychodrama Centre at North Walk, Lynton, North Devon, England)

HELMUT BARZ: 'GOOD THEATRE IS ALWAYS ARCHETYPE'

Jungian psychology and Morenian psychodrama can both lead people to rediscover something – in the first case, their religious dimension; in the second, their individual spontaneity and creativity within the group. In this perspective psychodramatic action can be experienced as fertile, fruitful terrain for the development of the individuative process, which is manifested in people's relationships both with others and with their own inner worlds. A more superficial assessment may have led one to think that psychodramatic action may be experienced as a way of coercing people to live through some forced collective social dimension that tends to negate their individuality. However, our research on Jungian psychology in relationship to Moreno's vision of psychodrama has been supported by the resonance our theory and practice have found with our colleagues from Eastern Europe and beyond. Concerning Jung's analytic psychology and Moreno's conception of man and woman, even our own individual analytical work makes us realize the parallels and common elements in their theory and, above all, the complementary nature of their practice.

This is yet another confirmation that individual analysis and group therapy can do nothing other than reinforce each other beneficially and fruitfully. Effective psychodrama must always be a piece of good theatre and good theatre is always archetype. Moreno's genius led to the creation of many innovative ways of working that can bring the pieces of an individual's life story can back to their sources – i.e. the archetypal model that defined their basis. In this way each person can instantaneously grasp moments of insight when he or she can recognize himself and find himself thinking again – 'Look, this is me.' Jung demonstrated that archetypes liberate a dynamic force that can direct an individual towards the total manifestation of his or her individual potential. This can happen if these archetypes – the collective models on which the kinds of behaviour of human existence are based – are investigated accurately and if their traces, even their smallest traces, are observed respectfully. Finally, Moreno and Jung were both thoroughly convinced that nothing radically meaningful happens in the life of the soul, understood as the psyche's deeper nature, that does not lead to an emotion that could ultimately be described as religious.

The idea is progressing, sometimes painstakingly, that Jungian individual analysis and the group technique worked out by Moreno are complementary. This idea is supported by the significant therapeutic effectiveness of a method that profitably unites two aspects apparently so different. This was immediately evident to our colleagues from Eastern Europe, who have approached our theoretical writings and practical methods with a fresh outlook and curiosity. In contrast, many therapists closer to home view themselves exclusively in the tradition either of Jungian analytical psychology or Morenian psychodrama and so still find it hard to synthesize the two.

Morenians coming from a unilateral perspective could, in the end, reduce psychodrama to a type of group therapy that has nothing to do with the unconscious and still less to do with the religious nature of the soul, something that Moreno himself considered very important. For their part, the least flexible and most dogmatic currents of orthodox Jungians run the risk of transforming analytical psychology into an elitist, esoteric, and pseudo-religious teaching interested only in the relationship between the ego and the unconscious, where an individual's belonging to a collective environment represents nothing more than an unavoidable bother. Both perspectives would lead to a profound misunderstanding of the spirits both of Moreno and Jung.

We need to be able to tap the reciprocal potential for enrichment deriving from both kinds of therapy and the conceptions of mankind they are based on. To do so, we need clear and reliable accounts from psychodrama group conductors with a wealth of experience who are inspired equally by Jung and Moreno. These would facilitate the fusion between the two techniques and help put it into practice. In other words, there should be books that draw their material from a great number of scenes enacted in real psychodrama sessions that can make evident the degree to which all the successful enactments can be interpreted as archetypal plays about the individual, the group, and the numinous. Such a kind of book is what we have here.

Wilma Scategni, a Jungian analyst, psychiatrist and psychodrama conductor, had the idea of making evident the parallel between Morenian technique and Jungian analytical psychology in a methodical way by employing a wealth of dream material taken from group members' dreams and enacted in the groups. Such dreams could be considered a kind of 'commentary' about psychodrama reflected out of the participants' unconscious. The idea proves to be as surprising as it is educationally fruitful. The author does not intend to formulate any theoretical speculation about Morenian technique or about dream work in analytic psychology. Rather, she is satisfied with letting the material talk for itself directly as it comes out of psychodrama and dreams. What she adds in her ample commentary and elaboration turns out to be thoroughly instructive for both forms of therapy. What happens to the readers of this book is that they do more than just revisit. They constantly see in new ways. They see depth psychology in the light of psychodrama and consequently they see the meaning of dreams in a Jungian perspective. Wilma Scategni has caught the spirits of Jung and Moreno globally and radically and has experienced their discoveries as real in her work. Thus what she writes about Jungian analysis and psychodrama goes for her own book as well:

> This is the way that the mythical nature of psychodrama and analytical work becomes evident: it gives everyday happenings more 'air' – more air to breathe – and enables them to flow into the world of the archetypes. The ritual in psychodramatic work may eventually cause the everyday – the here and now and the then and there – to be examined, to re-acquire its universal characteristics, to pass from some part of the universe into some remote place, and to change its nature from the personal to the more-than-personal.

Obviously, the author of a foreword wants the book he or she is writing about to have many readers, but I want something even more demanding than this. There should be many readers, but these should reach beyond the limited circle of professionals in this field. That is to say, there should be the sceptics – Jungian psychoanalysts wary of psychodramatic techniques and psychodramatists wary of anything that has to do with the unconscious. What matters is that these prospective readers again find just a little bit of their spontaneous curiosity and openness. If so, this book will prove as stimulating as it is useful for them.

(Helmut Barz is a psychiatrist, professor, and trainer at the C.G. Jung Institute in Zurich, where he has been president of the Institute's Curatorium for several years.

In Zurich he directs the Institut für Psychodrama auf der Grundlage der jungische Psychologie *[Institute for Psychodrama on the Basis of Jungian Psychology]. He is the author of numerous works on analytical psychology and psychodrama.)*

PETER SCHELLENBAUM: 'CROSSING THE THRESHOLD OF DREAMS'

The cadenced, repetitive and periodic rhythm that marks the holding of individual analysis and psychodrama sessions evokes an image of the cyclical nature of ritual itself. Rituals often serve to relate the mythical world of the gods, of the origins, and of the 'sacred' to the world of everyday experience and events. Rituals re-create – at least for a short time – the connection between earth and heaven and between the gods and the people, something that may have existed in a golden age. The passage from one type of reality to another is extremely delicate and has all the features of an initiatory experience. At least for a short time, this initiation opens the doors to the world of mysteries and the origins, to something that we can define in Jungian terms as 'the world of archetypes'. On the other hand, initiation sanctions the entrance of an individual into the social group to which he or she belongs.

At the same time, an individual's social dimension gets to be an integral part of the self. The ritual nature of initiation thus has the task of transcending the reality of the everyday world and taking a person into deeper and broader kinds of reality – those of myths themselves that relate to cosmogony. This happens when archetypal images come into play. Individual or group analytical work puts the outer world of the group and of social relationships into contact with the inner world of dream images, fantasies, feelings, and emotions. Thus this work is something like a ritual and hence easily fosters the blooming of initiatory images that take shape in dreams, in material belonging to the everyday life of the group that is brought into it, and in what happens in the group as an experience that is lived through.

Wilma Scategni's book takes up these themes as she illustrates and carefully analyses the great amount of dream and symbolic material that she delves into and scrutinizes with care and energy. The book is not only addressed to people in the field of psychology but those from the broader public who may be interested in the fascinating and complex world of the images that the soul uses in order to seek out its own way of expressing itself. It is written using fluid and clear language, even while it develops fascinating and profound concepts that have never been expressed before with such a wealth of nuance in Italian psychological literature.

A very significant and original feature of the book is its examination of the interaction of individual analysis and group work through psychodramatic techniques. The feature that joins the two techniques and guarantees that they complement each other is that very ritual aspect that has been emphasized. Working analytically on themes of initiation symbolism in a group context allows psychotherapy to free itself from the risk of a too narcissistic relationship with itself. Getting away from this dimension is a step that is indispensable in our times. In fact, the concept of initiation that the author addresses and explains helps us realize how a person may not close him or herself off from the outer social world in the realm of analytic and psychodramatic work when he seems to fold up into himself. Rather, he takes part in the innate forms of the human race. He makes contact with the archetypal images that populate his own inner world in a context that is not only individual but collective. This is exactly the key experience that psychodrama has led to from the time of Jacob Moreno. Psychodrama has used dramatic action and staging as a way of helping its individual participants blend into a kind of developing energetic flow. This energy joins the group and its conductor together as they live through a common experience that becomes a kind of resonance chamber sounding at every moment for each person.

It is exactly this shared experience that permits the 'Self' – that is, a person's own deepest and most authentic essence – to unmask itself as the real director of the scene that is played out in psychodrama in as much as it is an element that acts beyond the personality of the psychotherapist. What Wilma Scategni's work brings out in individuals is a kind of mysterious inner urge that starts to move and come out gradually. This is something that goes beyond any momentary projections onto the therapists. It develops as it evolves along the ego–Self axis – that is, the axis that links the conscious ego with its most authentic essence. This is the urge that gradually finds the room to come out into the open as much in the theatre of dreams as on the psychodramatic stage. When the underground initiation journey ends – as described in the section, 'The hidden treasure' (see Chapter 13) – the therapist fades into the background. Therapy as such dissolves and leaves room for individuals' natural vital processes to stimulate their potential for self-healing and bring it out into their conscious minds.

So it is that the object of the search is the Self – the very authenticity of a person. This is something that belongs to the symbol of totality, an archetypal value for humankind, which can be shared with the deepest essence of the group in the experience that it goes through together. At the same time the Self is something that belongs to the most intimate and unique values of each person's individuative path. Hence the issue is not to share abstract ideals, but to give concrete shape to the fantasies and images that express the essence of life itself. In this way, every thought, word, and image can find its own interrelationship, something that joins mind, body, and psyche together and so is able to transform the reality of the world in a concrete way. In this way there is no risk that words become meaningless ends in themselves that lose contact with the concrete nature of everyday life. All this is very well described in the section on the earth in dream images (see Chapter 12).

The themes in the dream take on a spontaneous development and evolution that go far beyond any verbal interpretation. This happens through dramatization. The group context opens the members up to the chance to let themselves go with the flow of feelings and emotions that the dream images may have evoked. These feelings are expressed through a complex language. Representing them involves all four psychic functions – intuition, emotion, thought, and sensation. The new consciousness that can be achieved is what I define as a kind of 'sensitive consciousness' or 'consciousness of the heart'. This is something that is much more multi-faceted and complex than rational consciousness. Psychodrama experiments with leaping from the inner to the outer scene and from the fantastic to the real gesture.

Dramatization of dreams and narrated scenes allows the group members to provide their fantasies about life with a concrete basis. It is possible to go on to concrete reality through the movements that accompany the words, which basically represent the gestures involved with enacting the scenes. The protagonist does not lie passively on a psychiatrist's couch describing and analysing dream images. Rather, he or she crosses the threshold of his or her dreams and follows the traces that the dreams have left, traces that take on a shape and a life with the therapist's and group's help. Even an anguishing dream can serve to re-orient, giving dreamers the chance to 'stay put' with their emotions and feelings while waiting to pick up on the transforming energies, however small, that would enable them to make out some 'sense', however faintly perceivable, or some direction they could follow in order to re-structure their consciousness.

The group acts as a sounding board that can amplify emotions, feelings, and perceptions and enable its members to perceive and gather in any elements as they emerge at every single moment – any new, minimal, and non-apparent elements that can become determining factors, any subtle potential vibrations of change. In this way it may become possible to explain a spontaneous impulse of healing in the place where it manifests itself and to make this impulse accessible to conscious perception. As said before, working in this way on dreams means entering the dream itself, as the protagonist does when he or she enters the centre of a psychodramatic scene.

This kind of entering the scene is a passage from narration to action. As such, it is often accompanied by uneasiness or fear in as much as it implies giving up what is purely private as well as what individual neuroses had comfortably been holding secret. The protagonist accepts becoming the centre of a transformation. At the same time, the attention of the other group members frees up a source of energy that leads all the participants to feel that they are deeply involved. In this way, they accept following the tracks that the dream suggests and giving the dream a form, while also accepting being immersed in a network of relationships that allows them to jump from the inner to the outer scene, from the fantasized gesture to the real one, and from solitude to sharing.

At the same time, protagonists experiment, act tentatively, and seek the ways towards new gestures and new psychophysical sequences of movements. They try to abandon behavioural shells that have already hardened and become useless and to make room for the seductive challenge of something new that is taking shape. They take up the challenge of trying something new that would let them turn their backs on the repetitive and stereotyped answers, the re-runs of the old familiar stories that had been caged inside. This is something like puberty or shamanic initiation. Hence entering psychodrama often activates archetypal images connected with the theme of sacrifice; the sacrifice – at least for a time – of one's own individuality, those features that are most closely linked to what Jung called the 'persona'. This occurs above all when the persona becomes static, hampers creative transformation, and forms itself into a neurotic shell from which a person merely observes the world without putting himself or herself on the line emotionally.

In any case, every initiatory passage is a transition rife with problems and dangers. In religious literature it is sometimes depicted as a narrow bridge, 'thin like a hair' or like the 'blade of a razor'. It allows the passage from one way of being to another – from one existential situation to a higher one with a higher level of consciousness. In psychodrama groups, the passage corresponds to overcoming the fear that often marks a person's real entrance into the group, emotional involvement, and regression. In addition, the group requires the sacrifice – at least temporarily – of a person's own individuality in order for him or her to bring meaningful events from his or her personal life into the shared space of the group and so to allow intense emotions, tears, and empathy to emerge.

It is worth people's effort to sacrifice these fictitious certainties in order for them to gather the fruits of their sacrifices. Protagonists in psychodrama groups can find countless facets of themselves opening up to be discovered before them, whose nuances and varieties they had never before been aware of. Each group member's inner images refract and reflect those of the others, strengthening and blending in with each other in turn, and sometimes opening up new paths. Thus each participant has the chance to meet up with and acknowledge his or her own 'personal mythologem' (their own specific 'myth' or 'story/history'), which is charted out in the very mythologem of the group as a whole. In this encounter, which is simultaneously personal and collective, the protagonists can rediscover the uniqueness of their own experiences.

Through sacrifice, sclerotic models of relationships gradually fall behind other, more flexible models that are about to be tried out. New vital potential that had been unknown before takes shape on the stage. The group and the therapist allow for amplification, resonance, mirroring, and reflection. In continuous transformation, these processes are a consequence of the fluidity with which the creative process of the protagonist's Self expresses itself.

Every dream that is brought to the group is the beginning of an unknown path for the protagonist and for the group, a road whose destination is unknown. Only some messages are sometimes partially decoded. Their constant enigmatic quality pushes the group members to continue a path of research that can never be entirely unveiled. The dreams that are dramatized and analysed in the author's groups have been chosen appropriately on the basis of this key to meaning. The dreams take on the aspects of initiatory rituals whose symbolism is expressed as dream images. In these dreams the protagonists sometimes go on journeys to the underworld and to the underground of the unconscious. Sometimes they go through the steps that are in common in shamanic initiation, such as dismemberment, visions, and encounters with the dead. They sometimes enter into contact with the basic elements of nature – earth, water, air, and fire.

This new type of post-Moreno psychodrama has been developed by Wilma Scategni, by the Zurich psychiatrist Helmut Barz and others. It represents an important evolution in Moreno's work blended in with the contributions of C.G. Jung's analytical depth psychology. Every conductor of a group should get to know this text as a way of reading more deeply into the relational dynamics of human experience.

(Peter Schellenbaum, Swiss theologian and psychoanalyst, teaches at the C.G. Jung Institute in Zurich. He is the author of Die Wunde des Ungeliebten *(Munich: Kösel)[The wound of the unloved] (1988),* Homosexualtät im Mann *[Male homosexuality] (1991),* How to Say No to the One You Love *(1992),* Der Tanz der Freundschaft *[The friendship dance](1993) and* Nimm deine Couch und geh*! [Take up your couch and go away!] (1988))*

Preface

This work offers some reflections on the appearance of archetypal images with initiatory symbolism in the dreams of analytical psychodrama group members. As I was working on this book, I followed the free associations that these images evoked and was not concerned about proceeding according to any coherent method. So, I do not claim to be formulating any theory or to be referring to any logical and exhaustive explanation of what has been happening. As I do in my psychodrama group work and individual analysis, I limited myself to putting out some hints that a person could eventually use as trail marks along his or her individuative path as he follows those images that could resonate inside himself most meaningfully.

This work definitely aims to lead the reader to listen to the echoes evoked by the material described inside herself or himself. I limited myself to letting memories and reflections emerge that were related to my experience as an analyst and psychodramatist. What I recalled made me focus on those themes involving deep emotions and feelings to the extent that they seemed to me to be the most meaningful.

Most of the dreams came into my memory relative to each research theme in a spontaneous way – often after many years had passed – because they were very intense emotionally. All the dreams treated here have been taken from my more than 20 years' experience leading analytical psychodrama groups and from individual sessions with patients who were simultaneously working with psychodrama.

My first groups originated in the public psychiatric service in local public health centres in Italy, where I worked for about 15 years as a psychiatrist and for more than 10 years as director of a district psychiatric station. I then continued this work in my private practice, where I worked with basic groups, training groups, and groups for the supervision of clinical cases that I conducted in the psychodrama training school of the APRAGI and COIRAG (both members of the International Association of Group Psychotherapy, IAGP). I also worked for the National Health Service as supervisor of *équipes* (health worker groups) and of institutional analysis programmes addressed to doctors, psychologists, and other workers in the mental health service. Other groups were and are now being held at the Jung Institute in Zurich and at workshops conducted during international conferences. Some are conducted by myself alone, some with a co-conductor. Some continuing groups – basic groups and training groups – run for 10 months annually. Others are limited to a definite number of sessions and resemble seminars. The participants are moved by a very heterogeneous series of motivations and expectations. There are patients from the public health service who are suffering from pathological conditions of varying degrees. They are motivated by essentially therapeutic reasons aimed at curing or lightening their symptoms. There are health service workers who are dealing with the nature of their place in their own profession, the sense of their practice. Their motivation is to receive training. Finally, there are group members moved by a desire for personal, existential research.

The dreams have certain themes. The dreams that I have written about were those with esoteric characteristics. I think it is important to emphasize that these 'esoteric' dreams were chosen from a very large body of material that was more involved with daily living and the problems of everyday life. However, these 'everyday' dreams are sometimes accompanied by the emergence of problems connected with the world of archetypes.

Some of the more personal and delicate details regarding the dreamers' personalities have been purposely left out in order to respect their privacy. The dreamers were also consulted in relation to material that concerned them. They recognized themselves coherently and gave their consent to have the material published. I owe all of them my deepest thanks for having made this book possible.

Wilma Scategni

Introduction

When the religious historian Mircea Eliade speaks about the difference between man in archaic societies and modern man in the Judeo-Christian tradition, he describes archaic man as essentially in harmony with the cosmos and its cyclic rhythms while modern man is someone who considers himself in harmony with history and its linear progression (Eliade 1963: 388ff.).

One of the problems of depth psychology is creating a connection between cyclic time and linear time in a person's experiences. In archaic societies, the cosmos is formed through a series of mythical events which, as it were, represent its structure. Such mythical events conform to the 'sacred' history as opposed to the 'profane' history of demythicized man. Sacred history can be repeated indefinitely. It becomes present again through the representation of myth in ritual action. Myths serve as models for ceremonies that periodically make grandiose events related to 'the beginning of the world' present, events that are transmitted through ritual. Ritual makes the creation present again by reactivating the energies connected to the event that 'belongs to the gods'. Here linear historical time, which sees man as a loser in the world of vicissitudes, yields its place to cyclical time – the world of transcendence where everything that is continuously destroyed is continuously re-created in perennial change. The symbol and the archetypal image expressed through ritual allow a person to pass from linear to cyclical time. Understandably, many primitive or archaic civilizations have used ritual for healing because ritual's regenerative power frees up energy (Eliade 1991: 63).

Contact with and re-immersion in primordial symbols allow individuals to participate in something that transcends themselves. Their chance to be born again comes out of their participation in the refoundation of the universe. The same contrast between linear and cyclical time – between the time of man and the time of the soul – can be found in the relationship between daytime conscious life dominated by rational thought and nighttime dream life, where the unconscious manifests itself through archetypal symbolic images.

The fundamental aim of the research of depth psychology is represented by the effort to harmonize these two aspects, to make the relationship richer and more dynamic between the conscious ego and the unconscious in its individual and collective aspects. This happens through what Jungian psychology defines as the 'individuative process'. In effect, the individuative process consists in a continuous relating and comparing of the conscious ego and its own unconscious contents – those of the collective conscious and of the collective unconscious.

This is made particularly evident in analytical work in psychodrama groups, where each participant is brought to measure himself and his own individuative process up against the conscious and unconscious expressions and contents of the group. Here within the *temenos* (ritual shelter) represented by the psychodramatic space, real scenes of life experiences alternate with memories and dreams that appear side by side. In the dreams and representations that are evoked, archetypal images emerge as they are being expressed in the iconic or symbolic aspects of the scenes that are played out. Their emergence unchains a transforming energy that privileges a continuous passage from the historical time of the 'here and now' of the experienced memory to the 'time of the soul' that the archetype dominates. Particularly, images or situations that go back to initiatory symbolism often appear in psychodrama groups. Initiation causes a person to transcend the reality of the senses and the everyday world and to create a bridge towards the consciousness of a sacred and eternal reality above the senses, the founding factor of existence itself. Psychodrama juxtaposes symbolic images and situations that free their intense transforming energy. The group gradually acts to catalyse this energy and gains access to a reality of images – the soul's reality.

The group may seem to resemble an esoteric sect with its own series of rituals and initiations. It forms a circle. It is the receptacle of all the projected expectations of the participants – hopes for recovery, nourishment, and regeneration, however ambiguous. Especially when a group works together a long time, it tends to create its own language, its own value system, and its own history, recognized as the expression of the culture of the group. So what turns up is a sort of collective conscious and unconscious of the group as a whole, with which an individual member can compare his or her own individuative process.

The analogy with initiation is strengthened by the fact that people who join the group for the first time can get the feeling that they are dealing with some kind of esoteric sect, to be entered only by passing some initiatory tests. Then the attitude of the group itself tends to confirm this impression. When new members act guardedly and mistrustfully because they have just entered the group, the group often takes an intransigent stance in judging them as 'not bringing enough of themselves in'. A group can be impressed by the sacredness deriving from its contact with a constellation of archetypal images and so can run the risk of taking itself too seriously and pushing itself towards mystical expectations that have nothing to do with everyday reality. The psychodrama technique itself sees to it that this does not happen, as long as it has developed the flexibility needed for rapid changes in direction. In fact, the most intensely fascinating thing about psycho-drama lies in its continuous character of transformation and in its rapid and continuous passages from the ridiculous to the sublime, from the comic to the dramatic, and from the moving to the grotesque. This is a characteristic of the dream itself. Analogously, all these elements often appear mixed up in an inextricable heap, rich with surprise boxes with hidden contents. All this works together to determine the continuous transformation of the psychodramatic time and space from external reality to the reality of the soul and, simultaneously, vice versa.

The group passes rapidly from apathy to enthusiasm, from empathy to disinterest, from *participation mystique* to the most absolute indifference, from irritation to intense emotion – through thousands of states of the soul. All this takes place in relation to the material that is brought into it to be seen. The evocative and emotionally charged material expressed in the telling of episodes from real life and dreams rarely meets with the indifference of the group. Dreams often carry emotionally charged contents expressed in a symbolic form. Symbols, the responses to conflicts that generate tension, carry a great charge of psychic energy and easily resonate with other archetypal contents. These are arrayed in the consciousness of the dreamer and of those in the group who are moved by the dream as it is narrated and enacted. The mobilization of psychic energy in the group is expressed in the form of interest and attention. In their ambiguity symbols allow people to withstand conflicts between apparently irreconcilable opposites. They make their way towards the consciousness in the form of archetypal images, push people to resolve their tensions in catharsis, and find their natural outlets of expression in dreams and in psychodramatic play.

However, it may sometimes happen that dreams that are apparently rich in meaning, when performed in the group, lose much of their symbolic meaning or turn out to carry no energy. On the contrary, it may happen that the enactment of apparently banal episodes may put out an array of archetypal images that resonate deeply in group members. If so, a great emotional charge is liberated in the group. In this way, a 'banal' episode may take on a strong density of meaning. In the same way, dramatic episodes that initially tell of the narrator's great emotion and anguish often are transformed as they are enacted into comedies that reveal hitherto hidden aspects. On the other hand, episodes and dreams that are apparently comic or humorous can be transformed in the dramatic play into climactic, anguishing, or extremely sad experiences.

It is also important to remember that psychodrama allows for more than one level of dialogue and reading simultaneously and that these manifest themselves over time as they find their outlets of expression. Communication takes place between the conscious and the conscious, between the conscious and the unconscious (both of the group as a whole and of the single participants), and between the unconscious and the unconscious in all possible directions. Some dreams arrange memories from participants' life experiences and vice versa. Other times dreams inspire dreams of response over time. All this finds its chance to manifest itself within the *temenos* of the psychodramatic space.

Part I

Space and time in psychodrama

Chapter 1

Psychodrama

HISTORICAL ORIGINS

The historical origins of psychodrama, like those of theatre, are hidden in the dark night of ages gone by. They are to be found in shamanic and magical rituals from different times and cultures and in the sacred dramas celebrated in various cultures. Anthropologist James G. Frazer relates that spells and magic ceremonies were used by people at a primitive stage of development in order to affect the forces of nature directly through human interference (Frazer 1922: 376ff.). In this way, they practised 'sympathetic' magic widely. It may be a valid hypothesis that the most phylogenetically archaic forms of dramatization consisted in representing the forces of nature themselves – the rain, the winds, the succession of the seasons, and the growth and decay of vegetation – in order to control their courses. The magic worked through imitation – that is, through the dramatization of natural processes that needed to be encouraged. Its aim was to obtain particular desired effects.

Frazer adds that these same effects were attributed to the energies of humanized deities who resembled people in that they were born, died, and married, thus determining the succession of night and day, of the seasons, of the rebirth of vegetation, and so on. In this case, the holding of the magic ritual could have the function of helping the god who is the origin of life in the struggle against the opposite principle that is the origin of death. This is what happens in the dramatizations of the struggle between Osiris and Set practised by the Egyptians (to be treated later). At this phase, the dramatic representation still focuses on the natural process that it aims to facilitate, according to the principle of sympathetic or imitative magic.

Subsequently the identification with the god through the ritual takes on the principal task of regenerating and re-awakening the energies of the celebrant him- or herself. As Mircea Eliade points out in his various writings, ritual offers the chance to transcend historical time through representation (Eliade 1965, 1969, 1974, 1991). It re-connects with the *illud tempus* – the time of the origins where creation began. The celebrant gets his or her energy from this very origin of creation. This is the point from which we can derive the use of rituals for healing that have been practised by groups of people from various origins and epochs. One of the most evocative rituals is one that Eliade describes – the 'sacred art of healing by sand' practised by the Navahos (Eliade 1991: 83–84).

The patient to be healed has lost his soul – that is, his vital energies and his sense of life itself. He is placed on a sand drawing that symbolizes the image of the cosmos and the creation. He is then covered by the sand itself. The sand drawing represents the twin heroes who are going down the path of benediction – the 'sacred path of the pollen' towards the dwelling of the heavenly father. The myth narrates that they reach their goal and then are initiated through the test of water and fire and the benediction of the sun. The therapeutic action derives from the immersion in the mythical time of the origins represented by the painting. (Subsequent chapters will deal with ritual healing.)

Rituals are dramatizations during which some kind of communication is activated with divinities or transcendent powers. They include the infinite variety of shamanic rituals of any epoch or culture, in as much as these communicate with *mana* (impersonal supernatural) powers of various origins. This is what enables the shaman to act as a conduit through which the people of the group or tribe obtain their healing energy. When rituals emphasize the struggle between opposing powers, they start to mean that they are helping the god who is the origin of life in his struggle with his antagonist, the origin of death. This phase of ritual includes the ancient Egyptian religious dramas of the struggle between Osiris, god of life and resurrection, and Set, connected to death and the shadows (Frazer 1922: 427).

Themes such as the struggle between life and death as well as the god's violent death and subsequent resurrection are common among the various gods like Osiris, who are connected with vegetation. These appear at various times and places, such as Babylonia, Phrygia, Syria, and Egypt. Thus fertile unions, death, and rebirth represent the centre of religious drama where magic and religion often blend together. Herodotus narrates that there is a lake in Seis in Lower Egypt near the tomb of Osiris where his sufferings were performed one night a year. The priests beat their breasts and thereby exhibited an exteriorization of sorrow connected with Isis's sorrow. They carried an effigy of Isis in the shape of a holy cow in procession. Lactantius mentions priests who beat their breasts to express Isis's sorrow and later changed their expressions to joy when the priest who was wearing Anubis's mask showed a lost child who has been found again. This is the god Osiris-Orus. What is a constant in the ritual is the expression of sorrow changing into joy over the resurrection of the god.

We can assume that analogous rituals were celebrated in various places in relation to myths connected with divinities linked with the vegetable world. These include the myth of Attis originating in Asia Minor and later imported even to Rome; the myth of Tammuz, who is alluded to in Babylonian religious literature; and the myth of Adonis, a derivative of that of Tammuz, known in Babylonia and Syria.

Mysterious rituals with initiatory characteristics often find their expression in public ceremonies – processions, festivals, and collective rituals – dealing with themes related to death, origins, and regeneration, which, as we have seen, are often connected to the rebirth of vegetation. Notice of these is sometimes marked. Sometimes relatively obscure fragments emerge, but often they are wrapped in the darkest mystery. The rituals linked to hermeticism and the cult of Isis that Apuleius discusses in *The Golden Ass* are examples of these rituals from ancient Egypt. The Eleusinian mysteries – so important in ancient Greece – were celebrated first in Eleusis and then mainly in Athens. They were linked to the regenerating influence on the vegetable and animal worlds. For long periods of time, they had been wrapped in mystery for the 'non-initiated'. J.G. Frazer writes that even the names of the priests celebrating the mysteries were forbidden to be pronounced. Inscriptions found at Eleusis indicate that their names were etched on bronze and lead tablets that were then thrown into the sea in order to safeguard their secret. The ritual centred on the myth of Demeter and Persephone. It consisted in the candidates' fast, their initiation, then a torch-light procession, and a night vigil. This represents the search that Demeter made for her daughter Persephone. Later, the communion with the divinity was intensified by the candidates' drinking barley water from a sacred chalice.

The essence of the ritual was kept secret by Greek writers who otherwise would have been committing a sacrilege, but it was disclosed by Christian writers. According to the second-century Christian writer, Hippolytus, the heart of the mystery consisted in showing the initiates an ear of wheat. Church father Clement of Alexandria (seconded by various modern scholars) relates that the centre of the unfolding of the Eleusinian mysteries seemed to be the dramatization of the myth of Demeter and Persephone. J.G. Frazer writes that the subject of the drama was the sacred marriage between Zeus and Demeter – i.e. between the male celebrant and the sacred priestess.

The cult of Dionysus can be considered to be more directly related to the evolution of the theatre – sometimes appearing in forms linked to mystery cults and sometimes to public performances. Like the previously mentioned divinities, Dionysus is connected with vegetation and the cycle of renewal. His cult was known in all of Greece, but was celebrated mainly in Thrace and on the island of Crete (Kerényi 1949: 186). Dionysus was known as the god of the vines as well as the god of vegetation, trees, agriculture, and wheat. As such, he shares in the themes common to the other analogous deities: he dies a violent death, is dismembered, and arises from the dead. His myth tells that he appeared in the form of a bull and was torn apart by the Titans. This is the episode that is referred to in the representation of the passion of Dionysus performed every two years in Crete. In it, there is a bull that represents the god himself as he is portrayed in some images and as he appears to his devotees in sacred rites. It is torn apart during an orgiastic ritual. The myth relates that tambourines and flutes had attracted the boy god towards a violent death. These accompany the sacred drama. The celebrants wander around the woods shouting frenetically. A coffer is carried in front of them that is thought to contain the sacred heart of Dionysus.

The scholar of classical mythology Karl Kerényi wrote that the most archaic forms of Greek masks were those of Dionysus and the Gorgones (Kerényi 1949:

193). Dionysus was the subject of a sacred drama in which masked dancers exhibited themselves and remained hidden at the same time. Rigid masks showing various expressions – tragic, comic, and satyr-like – were part of the great Dionysian representations of the Alexandrine era. A character often present in these representations is the masked Silenus whose goat feet signal his belonging to the nether world.

Kerényi relates that the mask itself without a wearer is an instrument of mystery that became a cult image. It symbolizes the presence of the god himself without the mediation of a human wearer. His presence in the woods and near fountains and tombs leads people to question themselves and hence creates the possibility of a relationship between people and god that makes the divinity himself present. The mask represents the quality of being in the world of men and at the same time of keeping a distance – a characteristic particular to the gods. In this way, the theatre takes on the apotropaic (evil-preventing) characteristic of a cult, a game, and a celebration all together. As a result, the dramatization evolves towards a mutual confrontation between people and gods, in which the people question themselves about what will become of them – something that is marked by time, fate, and death.

We can find the same dialogue between gods and people in the dialogue with the unconscious in the light of James Hillman's theory of psychology. The founder of 'archetypal psychology', Hillman suggests that mythology and psychology can be interchanged to a certain extent:

> The ancients had no psychology, properly speaking, but they had myths, the speculative tellings about humans in relation with more-than-human forces and images. We moderns have no mythology, properly speaking, but we have psychological systems, the speculative theories about humans in relation with more-than-human forces and images, today called fields, instincts, drives, complexes.
>
> (Hillman 1979: 22–23)

From this perspective we can consider that the communication with the unconscious expressed in analytical work is the relationship of the ego with the more-than-human powers and images that the ancients called gods. Thus psychodrama becomes analogous with ancient theatre and religious drama, which presents the events involving people in relationship with gods and those involving the gods themselves.

JACOB L. MORENO AND MORENIAN PSYCHODRAMA

Psychodrama as a therapeutic practice finds its expression in the work of Jacob L. Moreno. Moreno was born under extraordinary circumstances. It is said that he was born on a ship sailing on the Danube in 1889. He relates that he remained stateless a long time. He lived for long periods in Bucharest and Vienna, and only later became an American citizen. His lack of nationality was due to the fact that his parents were very young when he was born and were unable to fill out the forms needed to register his birth.

Moreno himself recounts the first psychodrama in his life (Moreno 1946: 2–3). When he was four years old, he found himself playing with his playmates in a cellar. He suggested playing the game 'God and his angels' since he was spurred on by his wish to play the role of God. To do this, the children piled chairs up on a table. Moreno took the highest chair that represented the throne of God. As his playmates were playing the roles of the angels, flapping their wings and singing, one of them asked him: ' Why don't you fly?' He then tried to fly and found himself on the floor with a broken arm. Moreno defines this the 'first private session' of psychodrama that he directed. At that time he considered himself director, patient, and protagonist.

This first experience brought forth the ideas of the multi-level psychodramatic stage and of the therapist as a demiurge who loves his creation. Moreno saw this god-like feature as the first manifestation of the idea of re-creating the world psychodramatically, something that was later to guide him. He wrote about the special shape of the stage in reference to his first childhood experience:

> The first inspiration may well have come from this personal experience. The heavens up to the ceiling may have paved the way towards my idea of the many levels of the psychodrama stage, its vertical dimension, the first level as the level of conception, the second the level of growth, the third the level of completion and action, the fourth – the balcony – the level of the messiahs and the heroes . . . That I fell when the children stopped holding up the chairs may have taught me the lesson that even the highest being is dependent upon others, 'auxiliary egos,' and that a patient–actor needs them in order to act adequately. And gradually I learned that other children too, like to play God.

Moreno recognized that he stayed committed to his image of the demiurge who loves his creation. This is exemplified even later when, as a student, he organized improvised recitals with the Vienna playground children. He saw the power of spontaneity and creativity in the children, which contrasted with the social stereotypes of the adult world. He writes about this experience:

> I permitted them to play God if they wanted to. When they missed, just as *I* was treated when my arm was broken, I began to treat children's problems by letting them act extemporaneously, a sort of psychotherapy for fallen gods.
> (Moreno 1946: 1–3)

On 1 April, the Viennese 'Fool's Day', in 1921 Moreno organized the first official psychodrama session in a Vienna theatre. Moreno's proposal was a free working out of the theme of the *Königsroman*. There were no actors, no script, and no plot summary. A velvet armchair with a golden crown on top of it similar to a king's throne stood out on the bare stage: 'The natural theme of the plot was the search for a new order of things, to test everyone in the audience who aspired to leadership and perhaps to find a saviour.'

Each person was invited to get up on stage and to act like a king. Between 7 and 10 o'clock – the length of the performance – no one got up on stage. The initiative was considered a clamorous failure by the press of the time. In any case, Moreno did not spurn his desire 'to re-create the world psychodramatically'. He recounts: 'I lost many friends, but registered calmly: *Nemo profeta in patria*, and continued to give sessions before audiences in European countries and the United States.'

His successive experiences led him to found an experimental theatre of spontaneous play on Maysedergasse near the Vienna Opera where amateur actors put on 'living newspapers' that represented the events of the day. During this experience, Moreno was very deeply impressed that dramatic play had a therapeutic effect because of the particular case of a young woman participant who experienced an intense reaction. This came about through the catharsis of the emotions. There was a young actress named Barbara who was usually shy and reserved in public. She was very talented at reciting roles as naive, romantic heroines. However, in her private life with her husband George – also an actor at the Maysedergasse spontaneous theatre – she exhibited an impulsive and violent temper. In the 'living newspaper', Moreno invited her to play the role of a prostitute who had been killed recently. He invited her to express her emotions violently. In the scene 'mild' Barbara cursed, kicked, punched, and shouted violent words at the actor who played the killer. The scene had a deep cathartic effect on the young woman, who said that she felt very relieved.

In successive encounters she often played the roles of choleric, vulgar, and trivial women. While this was going on, her private life took a turn for the better. Her fits of anger got shorter and less intense. Barbara often found herself smiling during these fits when she remembered analogous scenes that she had recited on stage. At this point Moreno brought Barbara and George on stage together to recite. The scenes they represented took on more and more the nature of their family fights. Gradually scenes were played out treating portraits of Barbara's and George's families, their dreams, and their projects for the future. Because all of this brought along a certain sense of immediacy, the audience members were affected intensely and felt that they were taking part more and more.

Moreno himself writes of meeting Sigmund Freud, the father of psychoanalysis, in 1912 and saying:

> 'Well, Dr. Freud, I start where you leave off. You meet people in the artificial setting of your office, I meet them on the street and in their home, and in their natural surroundings. You analyze their dreams. I try to give them the courage to dream again. *I* teach the people how to play God.'
>
> (Moreno 1946: 5–6)

Moreno tells that Freud looked at him bewilderedly.

The 'Theatre of spontaneity' soon became the meeting place and point of reference for those rebels in the field of classical psychology and psychoanalysis – fields that were considered too restrictive. It became the centre of a creative revolution. Moreno describes the rapprochement between psychoanalysis and psychodrama as a gradual coming closer. Some students of Freud were interested in the therapy of spontaneous playing with children – subjects who cannot be analysed in classical terms. The students then set up some situations where the children could interact directly with an analyst through games. The cathartic effect of this was soon recognized. Further, Moreno himself recognized that he was aware of the fact that he was living in the same city as a generation of psychoanalysts and that this had a certain influence on his work – even though he did not admit that this was positive.

Moreno later opened up a psychiatric clinic in Beacon, New York, whose work was focused on cathartic psychodramatic techniques. He worked on the training and therapy of actors. He became involved in re-education projects for inmates and girls with psychological problems. Doing this, he laid down the basis of sociometry – the study of the relationships among individuals in the realm of their interactions. Psychodrama remains the main tool of this field of research. Psychodrama allows people to free up their feelings through catharsis, then to gain consciousness of them, and to adapt once more to their interactions and social roles. In this sense, psychodrama takes on a 'pedagogical' function in the field of personal relationships, where a deeper perception and acceptance of other people emerges from the manifestation of spontaneity.

The first therapeutic psychodrama theatre was built for Moreno in Beacon in 1936 (Ancelin 1972: 17). Here Moreno activated the circular, multi-level theatre that he had remembered from his first childhood experiences. Moreno later committed himself more actively to psychodrama as a training instrument for doctors, paramedics, teachers, and educators. Sociometry became more and more widespread. Psychodramatic methods were used more and more in psychotherapy, pedagogy, and human relations.

During the first international congress of psychiatry (Paris, 1950), Moreno laid the foundation for the first international congress of group psychotherapy, which was held in Canada in 1954 (Ancelin 1972: 19). Subsequently, the first international congress of psychodrama was held in Paris in 1964 at the Salpetrière Hospital, the very place where Moreno had first presented the psychodramatic method 10 years earlier on the invitation of Claude Lebovici. In France, the psychodramatic method was introduced for child therapy in 1946 by Mireille Monod and for adult training by Anne Ancelin Schützenberger. Before that, during the Second World War, A. Charend, F. Tosquelles and M. Millon introduced theatre therapy and psychodrama in the psychiatric hospital in Saint-Alban (Lozère).

It is evocative to recall that in 1800 the Marquis de Sade put on some of his plays giving the secondary roles to mentally ill people. While he was interned in the hospice in Charenton, he suggested to its director that he wanted to offer dance and theatre for the patients – even though such initiatives were soon prohibited.

CARL GUSTAV JUNG, JACOB MORENO, AND 'JUNGIAN' PSYCHODRAMA

In her book, *Selbstbegegnung im Spiel* (The Encounter with the Self in Play), Elynor Barz emphasizes that C.G. Jung and Jacob Moreno were two essentially different personalities with deeply different life styles (Barz 1988: 13ff.). They never met each other in person during their lives. They never influenced each other. Yet, they met in theory through the later work of people in various currents of thought who were inspired by them. In fact, when analysts with Jungian training applied psychodramatic techniques, these techniques were the concrete expression of their reciprocal interest in Jung and Moreno as well as the evidence that there was a developing sense that their different typologies were complementary. This has made it possible for the two different theoretical matrices to co-exist, fuse, and reach a kind of synthesis. (Refer to the bibliography for further information on this topic.)

There is little known about any interaction between them during their lives. They lived almost exactly contemporaneously – Jung 1875–1961 and Moreno 1889–1974. They belonged to cultural environments which – if not common – were at least bordering on each other. Yet, there is only rare evidence that they knew of each other (Gasca and Gasseau 1991: 15ff.). We have some information about Moreno's knowledge of Jung – or at least, of some of his works – and about Moreno's opinions about them. Moreno gave Jung the credit for emphasizing the importance of the existence of a psychic substratum common to all people – the collective unconscious. However, he took Jung to task for not applying this concept more concretely in the setting of therapeutic group work or applying it in a more socially oriented intervention inside the collective reality in which people live and act. Moreno was convinced that this was the only way that Jung could have given a more concrete form to his theory of the collective unconscious. Contrary to the case of Moreno, no sources have been found evidencing Jung's comments or appraisals of Moreno's works. Nevertheless, what Jung thought of groups and their evolution is known.

Several sources cite evidence that Jung's disciples often found themselves embarrassed about this topic. Jung maintained that groups could encourage people to lose their sense of responsibility and independence, subject them to imitation, make them vulnerable to others' suggestions, and weaken the defences of the ego too much. Eventually, his negative attitude towards groups was modified and subjected to a re-evaluation. Subsequently, he held that the individuative path and the adaptation to the collective were a pair of opposites that nevertheless were able to become complementary.

In a letter written to the Los Angeles psychotherapist Hans Illing on 26 January 1955, Jung wrote that he had founded a group under the auspices of the Zurich Psychological Circle (Jung 1975: 219). At the end of this letter he confirmed the importance of group therapy and acknowledged that it could complement individual analysis. Jung recognized the possible limitations of both approaches. Group therapy could be limiting because it is collective and individual therapy could be limiting because it risks neglecting social adaptation. For this reason, the potential complementary natures of the two therapies emerge. Further convergence and parallels between the work of Jung and Moreno can be traced in the several matrices or influences that they share.

The influence of Socratic thought

In her book on psychodrama, Anne Ancelin-Schützenberger asserts that Moreno was inspired by Socratic maieutics (the 'obstetric' or 'Socratic' method) and Aristotelian catharsis, understood as a consciousness-taking and a purification of the soul (Ancelin 1972: 15ff.). Moreno begins with the basic assumption that everyone has within a creative thought that expresses his or her own individuality, something that can be likened to the image of the Socratic *daimon*. Just as Socrates used the maieutic method, a therapist should act as a 'midwife, an obstetrician' who has the task of delivering the *daimon* to the light of day by giving it a way of expressing itself. In *Daimon*, the journal Moreno founded, he writes of his own inner *daimon* who led him to look for his own personal pathway. In certain ways, the Jungian concept of individuation can be compared to this image of a creative thought that has the character of the *daimon*, in that this thought thrusts toward a way of expressing and realizing itself that is somehow connected with the image of a strictly individual destiny.

Furthermore, therapeutic practice was considered by Jung to be addressed towards the realization of the person and his or her own creativity through the individuative path. This is something that can be held to be somewhat analogous to Socratic maieutics in its vision of the therapist as midwife. The therapist fosters the coming to light of unconscious contents that allow the person to achieve and thereby accept his or her own individual destiny. The Socratic *daimon* can therefore be considered an analogue of the unconscious, whose power and independence are things that the conscious ego has to face up to. Moreno considered the function of the Socratic *daimon* to be closest to the deepest meaning of the term 'catharsis' itself, understood as the liberating moment occurring when the emotions are expressed directly. Moreno treats the concept of catharsis in Aristotle's *Poetics* in this way:

> Catharsis is for him not a primary but a secondary phenomenon, a by-product, an effect of poetry upon the reader or spectator. Certainly the early Greek philosophers and Socrates' Daimon were closer to the deeper meaning of catharsis although they had no name for it.
>
> (Moreno 1946: 14)

Jung does not use the term 'catharsis' directly. However, he compares the dream to a drama that is expressed and staged in a person's inner world (Jung *CW* 8: para. 561–64). The dream brings unconscious contents to express themselves directly to the consciousness. This effect can be considered analogous to certain aspects of catharsis.

The influence of Henry Bergson's thought

Jung and Moreno come together in a certain way in that they were both influenced by the philosopher Henry Bergson. Charles Baudouin points out that Jung is indebted to Bergson and to Bergson's influence upon his era because Bergson somehow sanctioned a liberation from the fetters of intellectualism (Baudouin 1963: 43ff.). There was a kind of rationalism and positivism that limited the vision of psychology when it imposed inflexible structures and rigid systems between the gaze of the observer and the immediate data of the inner world. As Baudouin points out, Bergson maintained in 1901 that the main task of the new century's psychology would be to research the unconscious. According to Moreno, 'To Henri Bergson, for one, goes the honor of having brought the principle of spontaneity into philosophy (although he rarely used the word) at a time when the leading scientists were adamant that there is no such thing in objective science' (Moreno 1946: 8). Furthermore, there are many other characteristics in Jung's and Moreno's work that can lead us to compare them more clearly.

Religious yearning

Jung and Moreno share a common religious yearning that runs throughout their works. Jung considered analytical work to be a journey carried out in the inner world in search of a meaning of existence, which he identified with the realization of the Self as the image of the divinity. For his part, Moreno is spurred on by his desire to bring people to their complete realization through the expression of their creativity. For Jung, the search for God is undertaken in completing and giving life to the images of the soul. It is the kind of search that was most fitting for Jung's introverted character. In Moreno, the search for God is set in motion by his extroversion. Moreno seemed to be deeply attracted to the image of the demiurge, the God who creates, and he identified with this in psychodramatic creation and realization. As mentioned, he put on the 'first psychodramatic session' in his life at the age of four when he aspired to play the role of God.

Basically, the path that Jung and Moreno took in their time represented a route of spiritual searching that offered an alternate to Freud's positivism, which was bound up in his rejection of religion. Moreno recognized and emphasized the importance of the great figures of religious history in the past and of the way they exercised a cathartic-therapeutic function in public. One might say that Jung recognized these religious figures as guiding lights and archetypal images that belong to the world of the soul and could perhaps be identified with the figure that he defines as the 'Old Wise Man'. This is an archetypal image that appears in dreams as well as in fantasies and seems to play a similar role.

Dramatic action

Jung recognized that dreams had a dramatic structure, outlined in 'The Essence of Dreams' (July 1945) and revised and amplified in the 1948 edition (as to be treated in the next section). He affirms that it is impossible to ignore that there is something like a dramatic structure in most dreams (Jung *CW* 8: para. 561–65). In fact, the dream can begin with some directions, a 'statement of place' where the protagonists are to be presented. Then sometimes there are time directions. For Jung, this part marks the end of the 'initial situation'. Then a second phase follows that Jung defines as the 'development'. This presents a growing complication of the situation that generates a certain amount of tension. What emerges is the feeling that something important is about to happen. Then we are at the third phase, which is that of the culmination or *peripeteia*. Here the tension is released and something decisive happens that affects the flow of events and determines a radical change. The fourth and last phase follows. This presents the *lysis* – the solution or result of the dream work that highlights a new kind of set up. By now the contents of the unconscious have come out into consciousness through the dream and have reached a new arrangement. The identification of these four points in the structure of the dream do not yet constitute its interpretation. However, they do allow us to trace out a script and a point of departure. In 'The Essence of Dreams', Jung writes: 'This division into four phases can be applied without much difficulty to the majority of dreams met with in practice, an indication that dreams generally have a "dramatic structure".' It may be said that the individual's inner world is the place where Jung recognizes the same dramatic structure that Moreno presents on the stage.

Dream work

Both Jung's and Moreno's work on dreams is strictly linked to the concept of dramatic action. Both maintain that the goal of dream work is to take the dreamer inside the dream itself. Nevertheless, we can say that Moreno gave dream work a rather marginal position in the total sum of his work. He confronted it only occasionally because he was more interested in work that focused on roles and on interactions between individuals. Yet, when Moreno works on dreams, he uses a striking amount of precision in reconstructing the scene. Before he enters the dream, Moreno uses the most exact precision possible to reconstruct the context where the dream takes place as well as the dreamer's mood, almost as if the presence of the sleeping dreamer were fighting with the conscious dream ego for the central role in the scene.

This brings us back to a concept that Moreno himself kept on asserting (Moreno 1946: 204). In fact, he affirmed that when a person is totally absorbed by a role, no part of his ego is free to observe this role and therefore to record it in its memory. (Moreno posits the problem of training the ego to fulfil the double role of thinking and acting simultaneously.) At the same time, the attempt to recall the most minute details both about the situation in which the dream developed and about the dream itself can set off a kind of 'warm-up' that allows the dreamer to experience the dream atmosphere most intensely. In this way, Moreno leads people to envision the dream according to its sequence – beginning, development, and end. Over the course of the dramatization, he invites the patient to live through his or her dream while at the same time being outside the dream as an observer.

In Moreno's work on dreams there is something about the associations made on the dream material that can be considered to be akin to what Jung defines as the work of 'amplification'. For Moreno, amplification is limited to what can be defined as 'stimulating the emergence of contents that are more pertinent to the personal unconscious' of the dream, without delving on a deeper level. This very interpretation of the dream can be more related in Moreno to what Jung defines as the interpretation of dreams on the 'level of the object' – that is, on a level that privileges an interpretation that is more literal and concrete than symbolic. The dream that Moreno relates in volume 1 of *Psychodrama* is an example of this. Moreno presents this as a classic in the 'theatrical interpretation' of a dream (Moreno 1946: 204ff.). We can notice how the interpretation that comes out of this is extremely concrete and refers solely to a happening in the past life of the subject.

The patient dreams of flying above the houses of his neighbourhood carrying a bundle in his arms that turns out to be his little sister, as he learns later through the associations he makes. What emerges is that he feels fear and realizes that he has a great responsibility that he does not feel ready to take on. The dream was related to one concrete episode in the subject's life that concerned his childhood: the protagonist's parents gave him his very young little sister to take care of when he felt he was still too young to take up this burden. Moreno's work attempted to bring the protagonist's feelings of resentment and anger towards his parents to light – emotions that could not have been expressed at the time – and then to help him work those feelings out.

In any case, Moreno ignored other eventual symbolic meanings of the dream as well as the possibility of its being interpreted 'on the level of the subject'. Nevertheless, the technique of dramatization itself calls for role changing and gives the dreamer the chance to play various roles. For this reason, it can be related to what Jung terms 'interpretation on the level of the subject', even if only indirectly. However, it seems that Moreno does not refer explicitly to this aspect relative to role changing, at least not in reference to this dream. Jung writes:

> Our *imagos* are constituents of our minds, and if our dreams reproduce certain ideas, these ideas are primarily *our* ideas, in the structure of which our being is interwoven . . . The whole dream work is essentially subjective, and a dream is a theatre in which the dreamer is the scene, the player, the prompter, the producer, the author, the public and the critic. This simple truth forms the basis for a conception of the dream's meaning which I have called *interpretation on the subjective level*. Such interpretation, as the term implies, conceives all the figures in the dream as personified features of the dreamer's own personality.
> (Jung *CW* 8: para. 509ff.)

What the visions of Jung and Moreno have in common is the knowledge that the final and deepest meaning of the dream is intrinsic in the dream itself, and that this is a secret message addressed only to the dreamer. It is something that can neither be expressed in words nor be subjected to any ulterior interpretation. Moreno refers to this as the protagonist's 'living through the dream in the psychodramatic action'. Jung refers to it as living through the dream through the moods, the images, and the emotions that emerge out of it.

THERAPEUTIC TECHNIQUE: FROM CATHARSIS TO THE WORKING OUT OF CONFLICTS

The psychodramatic practice that I am about to refer to represents a synthesis of Jacob Moreno's experiences and my own personal training as a group leader, which originates in C.G. Jung's analytical psychology and in phenomenology. The integration of these models has allowed me to graft a unique *Weltanschauung* or world view on to psychodramatic groups. Most of the groups meet once a week for 10 months from September to June. The encounters last two hours every week. The number of participants – with various combinations – runs from a minimum of seven to a maximum of 15. The participants sit in a circle, which marks the border of the scenic space. The group leader also sits among them when she or he is not busy at the centre of the dramatization. Usually – or at least in most of the groups from which I culled this material – there are two leaders. One has the role of group leader, and the other, seated at a table on the side of the circle, has the task of taking down 'observations' about the session. These observations will be delivered to the group at the end of the session. They deal with the themes that have come out in the session in relation to the path the group is following as a whole or to the paths of the individual participants, as the observer 'feels' them. As said before, the leader and observer change roles after each session. At present I conduct my continuing groups alone, assuming the double role of conductor and observer.

There is an initial silence that serves to beckon the group members to get themselves together. Then one participant, who may feel the need to, communicates his or her own experience. He or she may point out the presence of a conflict or a dream that he wants to understand better and to work out. The group leader leads him to represent the material that has emerged dramatically rather than to limit himself to talking about it. The episode in question – or a memory or another dream that has come up after making an association – is dramatized in the 'here and now'. Often it is the group leader, in agreement with the protagonist, who indicates which scene to play on the basis of the emotions that a certain scene may inspire as it is being talked about or on the basis of the emotional resonance that it sets off in the group. The protagonist chooses the necessary auxiliaries from among the group members and constructs the scene. In the scene, there are represented the characters, and sometimes, even the objects or abstract qualities that seem to be meaningful in the reconstruction of this scene. Over the course of the dramatic play, the leader may ask the protagonist to change roles one or more times. During the action, the leader may take on the function of prompter, standing behind the protagonist and expressing a kind of 'voice of the unconscious' that brings presumably unexpressed contents to light. Often the prompter has the protagonist's shadow speak and thereby brings him or her to face up to contents that are often in contrast with what the conscious mind expresses.

After the dramatization, those who have played roles and watched the scene express their feelings and emotions. In this way, they give back the protagonist's original material to him or her after it has been elaborated in this way. Other scenes follow the first scene. Sometimes they are evoked by the first scene, sometimes by previous sessions or material that has emerged in the flow of life outside the group. The material can be made up of recent events, memories that have come back to the consciousness, or dreams. At the end – roughly during the last 20 minutes – the observer gives back the material that has emerged in the session. When the leader conducts the group alone, he or she herself gives the final observations. In this way there is in psychodrama a constant coming together of moments when scenes are staged and moments when group members work out material in words. Thus moments that favour emotional catharsis are followed by moments of reflection (Gasca *et al.* 1988: 545–47)

The pieces of the group members' histories that emerge in the form of scenes can refer to their real lives, their dream lives, or even their fantasized or hallucinatory lives. The protagonist brings the group a formulation of this piece of life that becomes clearer through being staged. As meaningful portraits and scenes are represented, this formulation takes on features of the protagonist's personal situation and the group's that cannot be expressed in words. On the other hand, there are various elements that allow the protagonist to experience the same scene from different perspectives: roles can be freely distributed, the group leader can intervene, the protagonist can confront the other group members who are reciting the same scene, and characters can be exchanged. In these ways, the protagonist experiences the scene as part of a whole that has a sense in itself, in which she or he is simultaneously actor and director. Dramatic play is like the dream in that the dreamer is present as a protagonist but is also simultaneously 'experienced' through his or her own dream images that have their own autonomy. In dramatic play, the patient sets off and sets up the scene with the help of the group leader, but is simultaneously 'experienced' by the characters in his or her life and dreams as interpreted by the other group members. These come to life as they take on a life of their own within the scene. Analogously to what happens in dreams, one cannot foresee the emotions, the moods and the memories that will be evoked in the dramatizations. On the other hand, every protagonist gets to be an instrument in other group members' scenes. This happens when they play different 'roles' and at the same time 'put life into' the characters that they are assigned to play in the fragments of the others' lives. Ex-protagonists do this on the basis of the emotional resonance that these roles may evoke in them.

Thus the group lends out identities, costumes, roles, situations, scripts, environments, and emotions. Most of all, they lend out mirrors and a chorus that follow and comment on the action. Feelings, life histories, and experiences had first been virtually locked away inside kinds of 'private' worlds that differ in each person. These now become part of a common world as they are put up against two measures. The first is the expression in words – the story, the rational confrontation. The second is the scene as it is played out – images of bodily experiences, emotions, feelings, and memories. The group members are invited to play roles, to exchange roles, and to take part actively with their bodies and not only with the attention they may pay as listeners. They find that they are sharing in the experience of the scene in a very personal way. In this way a many-faceted vision of things appears like something seen through a multi-coloured kaleidoscope. This is something that is re-assembled from the pieces of the scenes that have been played out. These perspectives are expressed through the experiences and the ways in which the actors recite the parts assigned to them, in ways that are always slightly different from the protagonist's recollections (Gasca and Gasseau 1991: 26ff.). The protagonist has the final task of putting together the pieces that have been returned to him or her with the help of the group leader, finding out what they mean specifically within the history of his or her life's experiences. In this way the protagonist comes to recognize his own continuity in the midst of incessant change, finding himself in the centre of a transformation that involves himself, his fellow group members, and the therapists.

Analysis through dramatization uses fluid images that suggest different interpretative hypotheses in continuity with each other. These hypotheses have more than one dimension: they may be logical-conceptual, sensorial, corporeal, affective, emotional, and/or intuitive. Furthermore, these images are adaptable enough to particular situations specifically because they are at times created by the group members in relation to specific situations that they have faced. Therefore one can consider that the effect of psychodrama is not only based on the Morenian-type cathartic effect and the emotional-affective participation that this inspires. At a deeper level the effect of psychodrama takes us to analytical work on the inner world of the patient.

Putting on a scene creates this phenomenon: the 'subject' who decides to represent an event from his or her life – no matter whether it happened 40 years or four minutes before – is not the same 'subject' who had acted in the original scene. In this way, he or she experiences feelings and perceptions during the 'play'. Using these, he or she can compare the 'here and now' with the 'there and then' and hence can enjoy the distance of being an observer while not being cut off from himself or herself. Thus the individual can again have the chance to 'be a subject' as opposed to just an 'ego' determined only by circumstances.

PSYCHODRAMA AND THE DREAM

Jung acknowledges that dreams have a dramatic structure, as he outlined in several of his works (Jung *CW* 8: para. 509ff.). The sleep of the conscious ego and the rational conscience leaves room for the autonomous complexes to come out of the unconscious in their effort to express themselves to the conscious mind. Their allusive language is both evocative and fleeting and is expressed through images. The characters of the dream are parts of the ego itself and express its many-sided nature. All this allows for a double interpretation. According to Jung, there is the objective level – what the dream has to say about the persons and situations it is about – and the subjective level – the parts of the Self that appear and act in the dream. A kind of internal theatre of the psyche emerges.

Autonomous psychic entities that appear in dreams enter into relation with one another, interact, and transform themselves. The images that they bring out bear faithful witness to the process that is under way in the unconscious and give the conscious mind access to it through the traces the dream leaves on the memory.

Hermann Hesse paints an evocative and intense portrait of the 'Theatre of the psyche' in the last part of his novel *Steppenwolf* (Hesse 1963: 242). The protagonist finally finds the entrance into the 'magic theatre', but his ticket inside will cost him his 'brain'. In other words, he will have to give up, at least temporarily, his rational understanding. Here the mirror shatters where he had been looking for his reflection. In this way the man–wolf (conscious ego–shadow) dichotomy that he had been so familiar with is contrasted with the existence of very many pieces. In their infinite combinations, these offer him thousands of kaleidoscopic images of himself.

Jung sees an 'orientation to the setting' and 'a presentation of the characters' at the beginning of a dream, as occurs in plays and fables (Franz 1996: 37ff.). The 'exposition' follows, where problems are brought up that correspond to a modification of the equilibrium that existed before. This equilibrium can later turn out to show a further adjustment in the direction of reaching a new equilibrium that corresponds to a more developed order. On the level of the individual consciousness, the unconscious contents emerge, clear a way for themselves, come out into the light in dreams, interact, and transform themselves. In this way, they bring the conscious ego to a new way of structuring and redefining itself while going down the line of the individuative path. This is where the teleological and goal-oriented feature of the dream can be recognized. In fact, the *peripeteia* is followed by the *lysis* and the final resolution.

Thus Jungian thought accentuates the transformational meanings of dreams as expressions of their multiple meanings. It does this without letting the dreams fade in the light of a rational interpretation alone. Instead, Jungian thought leaves dreams with their own wealth of ambiguity and their endless ability to juxtapose images that keep on transforming themselves. As a patient's history is reconstructed, dreams often refer to events, images, and meanings that can be attributed to his or her everyday life. However, they more often refer to still more dreams, feelings, and archetypal images that evoke yet other images in turn. Just as the process of amplification goes on to find space in analytical sessions, it also goes on at an unconscious level through multiple and varied associative pathways that open up new routes.

The same thing happens in psychodrama, where a group's history may often be written out in dreams. This can express a kind of identity for the group, for the group members, and for their interactions. In psychodrama, there is a continuous interweaving of two dimensions – a 'thinking through images' and a 'reflecting on images'. This happens just as in dreams and in analysis. This reflection can be interpreted as something resembling what Freud defined as the 'secondary re-elaboration of the dream', where a more linear and organized structure of the dream is sought, something that unifies the pieces of the dream (Freud 1994).

'Reflecting on images' can also correspond to interpreting them, bringing them back into everyday life and seeking to grasp their causal and teleological meanings. After all, it may mean a rational approach. This is subtly intertwined with 'living through the images' and with seeking intuitions beyond the senses linked to a kind of esoteric quest. The levels of communication interweave here. A communication from unconscious to unconscious is associated with the more immediate verbal and non-verbal communication expressed through the body. Images bounce off each other, arrange themselves next to each other, and call up other images. What is created is what Hillman defines as an 'image space', where communication takes place through analogies and where the unconscious finds room to create its myths and make them live (Hillman 1979: 24ff.).

Just like dreams, psychodramatic play supplies a twofold potential for inter-pretation and amplification and this happens on the subjective and objective levels. The archetypal theme that emerges finds its resonance in the group. It is what determines the evolution of the sessions by sometimes changing their tack. In this perspective, the proposed play takes on features of a dream. If dream material is being handled, the proposed play takes on the reality of a 'dream within a dream'. In turn, the entire 'group session-dream' can take the shape of a dream of the observer about the material that has been evoked, which is given to the group at the time of the final rendering of the observations. As a result, the dreamer can some-times have the feeling that she or he has been 'expropriated' of her dream, that she has given the group her own dreams 'to feed on', and that she has found her dreams transformed or even distorted. With this risk in mind, it may be important for the dreamer to recuperate her or his own subjectivity in the group as her individuative moment. This moment is something that acknowledges the different features and messages in the dream itself and in the dream in relation to the group. The play-dream is therefore a moment of interaction between the ego and the other.

In this way the dream may sometimes be experienced as a sacrificial object that is 'immolated at the group' and the play that follows it can be experienced as disappointing. However, the sacrifice is able to evoke archetypal images that transform themselves. The sacrifice will turn out to be fertile if it creates the poten-tial for people to follow these transformations. On the other hand, there is the fact that roles can be exchanged. This is made possible through the 'use' of the other in psychodramatic play. This ability to exchange gives the dreamer a way to live through the dream in every aspect as part of a whole that has a sense in itself. The dreamer can offer himself or herself to the group from time to time as the actor-director of some scenes. At the same time, he lives through them but is also subjected to them in a perennial active and passive double role.

This is analogous to what happens in dreams, where the protagonist always has an active role but is also 'experienced' at the same time (according to Hillman's vision) as a passive onlooker of his own dream images. On the other hand, he will later be an instrument in others' scenes when he plays roles required for 'staging needs' and yet makes them active and alive on the basis of his own emotional resonance. This is a kind of 'being for oneself' that is found on the road of 'being for the other'. As mentioned before, the psychodrama group lends out identities, costumes, roles, situations, scenarios, settings, emotions, a chorus that follows and comments on the action and – above all – mirrors.

It is possible to have access to a magic door through which 'one goes out into another story' – even if only for a little time – the story of another person that is also a little bit one's own story. In exchange for this, one must be ready to lend out one's own clothes and armour, to put on other people's clothes and armour, to come on stage dressed summarily, and yet to sometimes be surprised to find oneself naked. It goes without saying that a person can sometimes feel a bit disoriented if he or she is travelling on a 'bric-a-brac' carriage (as one group member dreamed it) in a space that is sometimes very tight in the middle of second-hand clothes, used shoes, melodrama costumes, clown suits, cosmetic sets, jewellery, and flowered straw hats. With the help of the therapist and the group, the ego has this task: to recognize one's own continuity inside these endless movements – that is, to find oneself at the centre of a transformation that involves oneself, one's fellow group members, and the therapist.

Chapter 2

Psychodramatic space

PHYSICAL SPACE AND THE SPACE OF THE SOUL

In psychodrama physical space is important. The sessions usually are held in rectangular rooms. The participants are seated in a circle that traces the boundaries of the 'scenic space' at the centre. Thus they form a kind of image that can be considered analogous to a *yantra*, the sacred diagram that is described by Eliade (Eliade 1991:15, 1963: 397ff.). The space that is formed like this can cover the same ground as the archetypal image of the sacred territory – the *temenos*, or temple where the ritual is performed. The scenic space in this temple is reserved for the gods. In the psychodrama groups these gods are psychic forces, as James Hillman understands them (Hillman 1979: 22–23). This is the place where these gods have the room to express themselves.

Hillman maintains that the psychic forces that act within a person's inner world – instincts, impulses, or complexes according to present-day psychological terminology – can be compared to the gods whom the polytheistic religions recognized and venerated. As opposed to what he defines as 'the illusory unity of consciousness', Hillman asserts a kind of plurality of aspects, ways of being, and tendencies that move in sometimes clashing directions and that inevitably call the rational consciousness up to face them.

People once offered sacrifices, offerings, and rituals to the gods to placate their wrath. Similarly, the modern person with her or his consciousness is forced to cut some kind of deal with the forces that live inside him or her in order to win their favour, to unlock creative energies that were imprisoned, and to reach an internal equilibrium. The forces that dwell and move under the threshold of the conscious are capable of manifesting their destructive sides if they are ignored or forgotten. Individual or group psychotherapy takes on the function of an appropriate present-day ritual that does the job that rituals did in the past.

The mandalic image marks the boundaries of the centre, where the *axis mundi* (the axis of the world) is found. (We will treat this topic more deeply later.) This is the place where the shaman ascends to heaven and where the psychodramatic stage is found. In group members' dreams this is the place where, for example, magic trees and mountains rise up, where people bathe in baptismal water, where cadavers are dissected, and where there is a cauldron for brewing alchemical potions. The space that takes form from the centre and the path that is imagined there often lead to a long ascent along a steep path rife with dangers. The soul in its chaos can express itself inside the psychodramatic space. It can have its chance to take shape in the *temenos*, to set itself up around a centre, and to acquire a language that is to be articulated in many ways, but is expressed mostly through archetypal images and symbols. The group itself and the physical space it occupies become a *temenos*, a sacred preserve marked by a physical, emotional, and affective boundary. This is what Eliade could have described as a sacred space.

The priests and the celebrants do their ritual work inside the *temenos* or sacred preserve. Symbolically, they reproduce the sacred events of the origin that allow them to recreate the cosmos out of the primordial chaos. In this way, a hierophany (sacred ritual) is offered again. This is a ritual that puts a sacred event on stage and potentially transforms the space where it is held in a radical but temporary way. The profane space is transformed into sacred space. This allows the myth of the origins to live again in the minds and memories of the celebrants. The people assisting at the ritual – in their inner worlds – are thus touched in such a way that their existence may find its meaning again and be led back to the roots of its mystery. In other words, ritual causes a cosmos to be re-created and this cosmos brings along its own order and equilibrium. Just as the physical space of the *temenos* transforms itself into sacred space, the inner space of the priest and the celebrants undergoes a kind of 'sanctification'. Eliade maintains:

> Every kratophany and hierophany [appearance of strength and holiness] whatsoever transforms the place where it occurs: hitherto profane, it is thenceforward a sacred area. . . . To put it more precisely, nature undergoes a transformation from the very fact of the kratophany or hierophany, and emerges from it charged with myth. . . . In fact the idea of a sacred place involves the notion of repeating the primeval hierophany which consecrated the place by marking it out, by cutting it off from the profane space around it. . . . In this way the place becomes an inexhaustible source of power and sacredness and enables man, simply by entering it, to have a share in the power, to hold communion with the sacredness.
>
> (Eliade 1963: 368–69)

What happens in the realm of psychotherapy in relation to the search for equilibrium and inner harmony is somewhat analogous. However, it happens in a secularized way that fits in more with modern-day western mentality. The rational consciousness seeks to reach all of this, but hesitates to acknowledge the 'divine' aspect in it. In fact, in the light of the rational consciousness, the very rules of ritual can only seem to be requirements for procedures and order. However, the unconscious recognizes itself in ritual and so responds to it more deeply than the conscious mind. In ritual the unconscious finds the cyclical flow of circular time that is its own. The unconscious holds within itself the mythologems – the various pieces of a myth – that the myth alludes to. When the unconscious goes with the cyclical flow, its mythologems are freed up and set into motion. It can be said that psychodramatic space presents itself to its participants like a hierophanic space. Hence psychodramatic space becomes similar to the hierophanic structures of sacred spaces, as anthropologist Lucien Lévy-Bruhl describes them:

> To these natives, a sacred spot never presents itself to the mind in isolation. It is always part of a complexus of things which includes the plant or animal species which flourish there at various seasons, as well as the mythical heroes who lived, roamed or created something there and who are often embodied in the very soil, the ceremonies which take place there from time to time, and all the emotions aroused by the whole.
>
> (Lévy-Bruhl 1938: 183; Eliade 1963: 367)

Returning to the psychodrama room – something analogous to entering the 'sacred spot' – evokes leading thoughts, emotions, and dreams. Pieces of daily life mix in with archetypal images as personal mythologems are created as well as mythologems of the group as a whole. This happens in harmony with the analytic space's transformation into a *temenos* during the sessions.

The fact that interior space has been restored its sacredness can be considered an achievement of Jungian psychology, which transformed the space of rational understanding into the space of the soul. In Jung's psychology, 'understanding' has still remained a factor to be accounted for, but it means much more than simply 'rational knowledge', something whose limitations are acknowledged. Jung's is an empathetic and intuitive understanding that is less clear-cut but more all-inclusive than rational knowledge. It ultimate goal is to harmonize the individual with his or her own inner space, and through this, with the cosmos and his individual destiny.

The modern world is relatively free of 'sanctified spaces', or at least of spaces that feel like this. In this context, the space for analytical reflection is a space for silence and for listening to people's own voices and inner images that can be taken for a sacred space, a theatre where people's *daimones* create and present their own personal mythologems.

The space takes life and tends to organize itself around a centre. It is made alive again through ritual. A person inside this space will have the images of his or her soul come alive again. This space becomes alive just like the space in the archaic world that Lévy-Bruhl discussed. Forgotten dreams and memories return enhanced by new memories or fantasies. In this way, the room where the group is gathered gradually takes on new meanings. It is symbolic space and space that is really being experienced at the same time. As such, this space appears enriched and transformed in the group members' dreams. Their inner images come out here. They face each other. They interact and create new ways of speaking in the space that may be said to be 'consecrated' by the repetitive ritual nature of this time and space. These images evoke other images and sometimes progress towards people's working them out rationally. As in theatre, in psychodrama groups the repetition of ritual is only partial. There is the steadiness of the space, the regulated rhythm of the time, and the representation of some symbols – the circular arrangement of the group members and the scenic space at the centre. This set of circumstances allows the conscious and the unconscious to express themselves creatively and simultaneously. This happens in a way that is consistent and repetitive as archetypal symbols emerge and make their appearance in an infinite variety of ways. The images that appear like this recapitulate the transformations of the individuative process in a myriad of ways, just as happens in fairy tales.

The unconscious in the group works analogously with sacred space. Once the unconscious frees its own energy, and once this energy is channelled and gathered in again by the individual group members, they emerge from each session enriched by stimuli and questioning. This process causes an inner movement to emerge that renders the participants more open to the potential for transformation.

Only a very well defined zone makes contact with the sacred possible. A moment of fundamental importance for the sanctification of space happens when external or profane space is 'fenced off' and zoned out. Eliade writes:

> The enclosure, wall, or circle of stones surrounding a sacred place – these are among the most ancient of known forms of man-made sanctuary. . . . The enclosure . . . also serves the purpose of preserving profane man from the danger to which he would expose himself by entering it without due care. The sacred is always dangerous to anyone who comes in contact with it unprepared, without having gone through the 'gestures of approach' that every religious act demands.
>
> (Eliade 1963: 373)

This is the reason why psychodramatic space, which is analogous to analytic space, is a 'protected' space. A person can enter this inner space only after 'preparatory rites' consisting in the questions of those aspiring to take part, the therapist's examination of the motivations, and a waiting period. All this precedes the acceptance into the group.

The marking out of the space also functions as a double defence – from the 'outside' and the 'inside'. It is a defence from the outside just like the walls of a city. It allows people to outline an area, or a perimeter inside which there are no intervening forces or foreign influences, where feelings, thoughts, and emotions can emerge in a chaotic form, settle, take shape, and express themselves. This is a process that leads from chaos to cosmos. Similarly, the marking out of the space – the *temenos* – is a defence from the internal. This defence is activated at the moment when the *daimones* that were called up – that is, the forces of the unconscious – are blocked in, fenced off, and contained. This process allows them to be reflected, channelled, and reworked within the context of the group. At the same time, the group holds in the destructive forces, allows them to show themselves, and frees up the energy locked inside the complexes by giving them the chance to be expressed and worked out.

SYMBOL AND ARCHETYPAL IMAGE AS GATEWAY BETWEEN PHYSICAL SPACE AND THE SPACE OF THE SOUL

With the fencing off of what we have defined as a kind of sacred space, symbols appear that are represented within the group. They are arrayed side by side or appear one after another as multiple archetypal images. These symbols serve as the gateway between physical reality and the so-called 'reality of the soul'. Psychodrama groups usually meet in square or rectangular rooms, the general form of rooms in present-day buildings of our time, but nothing stops them from holding sessions in other kinds of architectural spaces. The arrangement in a circle was originally chosen for essentially practical reasons. A circle allows each participant to be and to feel equally distant from the centre and lets everyone see the others and be seen, something like the round table of King Arthur's knights. A circle inscribed in a rectangle outlines the structure of a *yantra* or cosmic diagram. This is something that often appears in the group members' dreams. Here is an example:

> It is evening and I find myself in Piazza S . . . [a square where the room in which the group usually meets is located]. The city is deserted. I realize that other people are coming up to me in the square. There are five of us in all. I recognize other members of the psychodrama group. We arrange ourselves in a circle with the feeling that we are waiting for something. Five balls of fire come down from the sky and fall down at our feet marking off a pentagram.

As is known, the circle is a symbol of the Self. As such, it has assumed a basic importance in the magical and religious symbolism of various epochs and cultures. The circle sometimes appears in group members' dreams with these same connotations, at least in connection with the experience that is alluded to here. In *Patterns in Comparative Religion*, Eliade writes that in tantric symbolism the *mandala* or circular form is simultaneously an *imago mundi* (image of the world) and a 'symbolic pantheon' (Eliade 1963: 373). The word *mandala* is translated into Tibetan by an expression meaning 'centre' or 'that which surrounds'. The images of various tantric divinities are represented within this circle (whether inscribed inside a square or not). The initiation of the novice essentially consists in his or her penetrating the various zones or levels of the mandala. A diagram of the mandala is drawn on the earth with coloured thread or with coloured flour or rice.

Analogously, a group member seeks his or her own centre of inner balance as he or she moves inside the circle in all possible directions and meets the 'divinities' or the psychic forces and entities in the sense that Hillman understands them (Hillman 1979: 22–23). These forces are the participant's own forces or those of the others. In any case, he or she faces up to them through the many interactions that are possible. The participant feels protected by the 'magic circle' of the group, just like a city dweller inside the walls of a city. At the same time, the group exhibits the features of a labyrinth and a magic spiral. It is a labyrinth in which a person can perhaps encounter his or her own unknown visitors and monsters as well. If one finds the centre, the shamanic ascent is possible.

As an archetypal image, the symbol is an opening that allows one to pass from one state of being to another and from one existential situation to another. The symbolic image expresses the archetype. The archetype takes on the function of a threshold, a two-faced Janus (the Roman god of gates) that looks towards the spaces of the world and the soul. The tension between these opposites and the difficulty of the passages are expressed in initiation symbolism as a 'narrow passage' or a 'dangerous bridge'. Iranian mythology tells of a bridge that can be as straight as a razor's edge. It is the bridge Tschinvat, which the souls of the dead cross in their voyage after death. The early Christian *Vision of St Paul* alludes to a bridge as 'narrow as a hair' that connects our world to paradise. This same image is found in Arabic mystical writers. The passage across a narrow opening is at the centre of many initiation rituals.

What this corresponds to in psychodrama is the fear of 'really' entering the group, the fear of letting oneself go in a regressive space, and being submerged in a world of shadows that is no longer controlled by the consciousness. These are the same fears that are easily found in people that set forth on an analytic path and/or individual analysis. At this time the group space can be felt as something threatening, as is seen in some of the dreams that are examined in the next chapter. The theme of the so-called 'building sacrifice' can be linked to this theme of fear. A building sacrifice is required for the marked-out space to become a 'sacred space'. Eliade attributes this to a symbolic imitation of the primordial sacrifice in which the world originated (Eliade 1991: 30). This cosmogonic myth that appears in various cultures explains the creation by positing a killing of a giant (Ymir, Purusa, and Pan Iku in Germanic, Indian, and Chinese mythologies respectively). Such a cruel sacrifice is required to re-create the cosmos from chaos. This is something that is repeated in every building project (a house, a temple, or a *temenos*). For such a construction to last, it has to be animated by this sacrifice. Themes like this often recur in ethnology and folklore.

In psychodrama, the profound and 'real' acceptance by the group itself can be considered to be an entrance into 'sacred space'. The price of this entrance is 'the sacrifice', at least temporarily, of one's own individuality in order to participate in a shared space. At times, initiation and baptism are talked of as moments that set off a deep involvement. The group asks for 'blood and tears', it is said. The emotional entrance into the group is marked by meaningful events in the participant's life history that are brought into the group and dramatized. These give forth feelings, tears at times, and intense empathy. Similar episodes often give the participants a sense of 'belonging' to the group. Often a deep sense of trust and acceptance emerges. The centre is another symbol that often appears and is expressed on many occasions in various dreams referring to the group centre. As we have seen, the centre of the mandala is the place where the altar is built that is the starting point for the re-creation of the cosmos from chaos.

The 'psychodramatic space' is inside the circle located at the altar. This is the place where the 'gods of the unconscious' are granted the right to live their own lives. Images clearly linked with initiation often appear in group members' dreams – images of the *axis mundi* (shamanic trees, sacred mountains, and magic ropes). The *axis mundi* can be understood as a kind of 'cosmic axis' that various primitive cultures recognized – that is, an axis that passes through the centre of the world, serves to connect the earth, the heavens, and the underworld and allows energy to circulate freely across these three levels. It also serves as the reference point or base on which the world and the cosmos are structured. When psychodrama group participants look to find their own 'centre' in group work and analysis, they are looking for their own *axis mundi*. This is the meaning of their own lives, the reference to the self that can serve as their basis for reconstructing a cosmos from their emotional chaos. It has a meaning, gives meaning, and puts the pieces of their existence together. Hence group work takes on the feature of a double quest for one's 'personal centre' and for the 'centre' of the group. These centres are sought out for their stability and changeability at the same time.

Perhaps one can say that psychological space 'becomes holy' when it is transformed into a space for a participant to listen in. Here the conscious ego does not claim to 'understand rationally' and leaves space for the receptive, the passive, the permeable, and the flexible. In such a situation, what Jung defines as 'the little people' – images and phenomena that emerge out of an archetypal space – are able to be experienced. Eliade's image of the *temenos* in which the celebrant re-creates the cosmos from chaos may bring Moreno's guiding idea to mind – what he jokingly defines as his desire 'to re-create the world psychodramatically'.

PSYCHODRAMATIC SPACE AS IT APPEARS IN GROUP MEMBERS' DREAMS

The dramatic space that we have described often recurs in group members' dreams, appearing in many different transfigurations that address the themes described above. The following dreams to be looked at will be accompanied by only a brief interpretative comment or reference to their real-life situation to avoid the confusion that such an abundance of material may bring and to let the dream images speak for themselves.

> They invite me to a party, but when I go inside the house, I find myself in a big room where people dressed in white are walking. I recognize some of my fellow group members who pass me by without seeing me. I realize that they have spots on their faces even though it seems to be a natural thing for them. I feel uneasy and I am afraid of contagion.

The dream was brought in by a participant a few months after he entered the group. It expresses the idea of the space experienced in psychodrama as a kind of gateway. The dream clearly emphasizes a fear of suffering in the participant that the group may have transmitted to him. In the dream the unnerving side of entering the 'space of the gods' predominates, while its positive potential has not yet been recognized. The participant's motives for joining the group were mainly professional. He chose psychodrama for its 'play' aspect. His dream reveals and accentuates the other aspect of psychodrama – its disquieting aspect. This is something that he had already experienced in the group. Its evolution into something positive came out in his associations and subsequent dreams. When he went over his thoughts after the dramatic enactment, he said that he felt that there may be a better chance for him to heal himself more permanently in that very context, no matter how unnerving it may be. However, this potential was hidden somewhere inside the room and had to be looked for.

The following dream uses images significant for bringing out the theme of the transfiguration. In it, a space for regression and fusion is transfigured into a space for individuation.

> The group is in a barn-like room. It is nighttime and there is a lamp in the middle of the room. The light reflects a shining circle onto the floor. At first it seems that there is nothing inside. Then I notice that there is a very intense life among the insects and gnats there. After this the group leaves the room and everyone goes his own way. It's snowing outside. Gigantic snowflakes hit me. I note their harmony and symmetrically crystalline structure.

After the dream was enacted, the participants realized that the group space first appeared in the dream as a place of welcome where they had the chance to warm themselves among the herd that they belonged to. The circle of light at first seemed empty, but later it was seen as teeming with life. It was associated with the relations among the group members that had first seemed to be non-existent but later turned out to be rich in interpersonal dynamics and mutual interests. However, the barn's aspect of regression and fusion seemed to serve as a prelude to the required task of facing the cold, that is, the solitary individuative path out in the open, where each person went his or her own way. In this dimension it was possible to appreciate the symmetrical harmony of the snowflakes, even if only fleetingly. Their unity and perfection were associated with the loneliness of the individuative path and the symbol of the Self.

On other occasions, psychodramatic space appears as a means of transportation for a trip.

> In the central square of the town where I lived as a child there is a minibus that I see members of my psychodrama group get on. I follow them and get on. I notice that the sign that is supposed to show the destination is completely blank. The bus driver is wearing mountain clothes. He is someone I don't know. While I am wondering if the group is going to meet or not, I notice that the bus is going towards a snowy mountain.

Here the psychodramatic space becomes a means of transportation, a 'going towards', a starting off from one's home town towards a goal that the group shares. The sign for the destination is blank. This seems to indicate that it is not possible to define the goal ahead of time or to identify it with something concrete that can be written down in 'black and white'. The bus driver is the only one who may know the destination of the trip. He is an unknown but seemingly well equipped. Perhaps he is a personification of the 'transcendent function' that is activated by analytic work.

This dream takes up the same themes of travel and psychodramatic space as travelling space:

> I am riding in a compartment in a train with some other members of my psychodrama group. C. gets in at a little country station. [C. is another group member.] C. brings me an old suitcase that I had thought I had lost a few years before. It holds a lot of personal effects and also some things that may be rather compromising. The same scene repeats itself several times in the successive stations with other group members.

Simply by being present, the other group members allow the dreamer to reclaim pieces of his history and inner reality, something that the lost and found suitcases seem to be alluding to. Travel and psychodramatic space as transportation seem to be associated thematically with a person's search for his or her inner and social identity, as in the following dream (to be treated more extensively in the section on transvestitism).

> I find myself on a trip with the psychodrama group on a horse-drawn wagon that has all the features of a circus wagon and of a knick-knack cart. In the middle of it there are old and new clothes of all styles and sizes, used shoes, costumes from melodramas, clown suits, make-up equipment, jewels, and flowered straw hats. I notice I have only my underwear on and at first this creates a certain uneasiness in me, but bit by bit I realize with satisfaction that this will let me put on everything more freely.

Here psychodramatic space is again a means of transportation directed towards an unknown destination. The group members are caught between the serious and the facetious. They seemingly question their exterior identities as 'social persons', represented by the clothes and by the chance they have to swap clothes and even to jokingly cross-dress. They question their deeper and more vulnerable essences, represented by the underwear.

In the same group member's dream, which follows, the group transforms itself into a steady, welcoming space. This may have to do with the issue of integrating the shadow into the group – the black cooks and waiters who provide the food.

> Around the corner from my house I discover the presence of a sort of Grand Hotel that I had never seen before. I have the impression that this thing has

something to do with me and I enter the hall. I recognize some group members who are chatting with each other and eating holding plates. I notice several waiters in livery with dark skin. One of these comes up to me and offers me some very delicious-looking and nourishing food. I then notice a door opening to the kitchen and I observe that the cooks are also black.

In conclusion, we will consider some dreams about psychodramatic space that were dreamt by training-group participants. These people had already completed a formal educational programme as well as two or more years of group work on themselves as patients. By that time, they were aspiring to become psychodramatists and to put themselves to the test as group conductors.

> The group is seated at the edge of a kind of great round tub made out of some sort of rough material. I am happy to see that R. is there too, who is wearing a ring in an ear. The tub is a kind of pool with water inside. The woman group leader is wearing gypsy clothes and throws us into the tub one by one, saying 'Ready . . . Go!' and keeping the time with a stopwatch.

Here the dramatic space is a tub where the members learn to swim. The material that the tub's container is made of is a richly authentic 'raw material'. The group leader's gypsy clothes refer to a previous dream of B., another group member. B. had been in the group for a long time and played the role of a guiding figure for the dreamer, a young woman psychologist. B.'s dream had involved a group of dwellers of a land over the border who had rediscovered their common ethnic roots. This land is another example of a commonly experienced space and the theme of 'rediscovery' of roots, analogies, and memories is what came out of the psychodrama.

A young doctor brought in this dream on the eve of his first experience as group leader:

> I find myself in an amphitheatre. W. and M. [the psychodrama group leaders] accompany me to the centre of the room and then they wish me good luck and leave. I then realize that the group members are in front of me. They are looking at me inquisitively.

Several group members associated the room with the medical school amphitheatre for the introductory anatomy classes where cadavers were dissected. The dreamer found himself here again as if he were in medical school. He had to demonstrate that his ability to observe and his acquired skills were enough to transform theory into practice. The stance of the departing group leaders alludes to the fact that the time was ripe for him to take up his responsibility.

The same doctor brought in another dream right before he was about to conduct a group himself for the first time.

I am in a space where there is a lake in the middle. I see my girlfriend in the water. She is swimming but seems to be in trouble. I realize that I'll have to make an effort to bring her to the shore. I then notice that I have a doctor's white smock on and that I have to take it off before I jump into the water.

This dream seems to be saying that it is possible for him to conduct a group only if he is ready to take off his professional uniform (the white coat) – at least temporarily – so that he can save his anima (his girlfriend) as a figure to guide him.

Chapter 3

Psychodramatic time

HISTORICAL TIME AND THE TIME OF THE SOUL

Psychodrama takes place at real times, with sessions repeated at regular intervals, just like individual therapy sessions. Usually the sessions are weekly and last two hours. The time evoked and experienced in psychodrama can be said to belong to three different dimensions and can be seen from three different perspectives. The first is the dimension of the 'here and now' – that is, the moment experienced during the course of the sessions. The second is that of the 'there and then' – that is, the dimension of the memory which lives again by being evoked. The third is the timeless dimension of dream. These three different perspectives or dimensions criss-cross each other continually, so to say. They blend together and then stand out singly to express their characteristics during the course of the sessions.

The time of the 'here and now' is the time experienced at the moment among the participants of the group, between the group as a whole and its leaders, between the leaders and the individual members of the group, and between one leader and the other. This includes all the possible interactions, which come forth in the dynamics, the transferences, the countertransferences, and the collateral transferences present. Even in this time dimension, the other two dimensions – memory and dream – are constantly being brought to the fore by the people who are present themselves and by the more subtle interactions among their relative personal unconsciouses, those of the group as a whole and those that are collective. In this way the interactions go down a myriad of pathways. Only some of these interactions come into consciousness quickly and clearly. Others go on undisturbed and reveal themselves only much later in the group's history, when they emerge only partially or emerge transformed by their journey. Others proclaim themselves as clear answers to questions posed long ago in time, and other interactions do not come forth at all. Beside this, there are the dreams that can express a group history that follows its own path. There we can find 'dreams in response' that often express relationships of transference, countertransference, and collateral transference.

The second time is the time of memories and of the memory. Events from the lives of the participants – no matter whether they happened a few seconds or many years before – are reported to the group and played out there. The playing out and subsequent reflection on it allow the participants to see themselves over time. Hence they can recognize that they are partly the same and partly different. They can contrast the 'here and now' with the 'there and then' in their states of mind and in the experiences evoked by the scene itself and by their memories. Memories are also not unchangeable, but can be transformed and can sometimes evolve. Memories often change faces and profiles as they are viewed from differing perspectives. All this makes memories more 'subjectivized', more transformable, and hence more pliant to elaboration. When a person enacts memories – as happens with dreams – he or she may become able to feel which aspects of his or her memories have kept on living, stirring, and giving out energy and which aspects have seemed to fade into the distance and go out. As the pieces of emerging memories are enacted, they allow the group to win back their own personal lives. In fact, they have the chance to stitch together their own histories and to try to identify their own personal myths and to let those myths live in the group. The role-playing and exchange suggested by the group leaders allow the members to see differing perspectives. Thus 'personal myth' is enriched by variation and flexibility.

Dreams are associated with memories and take on the same psychic reality in the group as memories of daily life experienced in fact. The archetypes implicit in the roles may uncover roles lived out in everyday life, roles assigned by the projections of the other members of the group, and roles suggested in the scenes that are played out. In this way the third above-mentioned time dimension comes into play. This is the time without 'duration', the atemporal dream space that negates time as linear continuity.

The expression of the ego and of the personal unconscious finds some room in the roles that are being played out. Here emerge the 'complexes of affective tonality', as defined by Jung. The complexes of affective tonality, or 'autonomous complexes', are contents of the personal unconscious that evade the control of the consciousness. Their manifestations often take on the characteristics that contradict and clash with the consciousness itself. These complexes are mostly related to problems strictly linked to the personal life and the life of relationships of the subject. When these complexes show up and burst into the consciousness, they carry a charge of energy that often makes them come along with intense emotional outpourings. These complexes emerge with a certain ease and are often unmasked in psychodramatic play.

As the personal unconscious is being expressed, the 'complex of affective tonality' is dominated and influenced by that archetype which corresponds to it in the realm of the collective unconscious. The archetypes are structures related to that deep level of the psyche that Jung defined as the 'collective unconscious'. They represent a kind of innate disposition to produce symbols, a disposition that is part of the very structure of the psyche. According to Jung, this disposition is analogous with those instincts in biology that determine definite patterns of behaviour. Archetypes appear by producing mental images, which he defines as 'arche'-'typal' images (i.e. etymologically, 'commanding' an 'image', 'imprint', or 'seal'). These constitute a sort of collective patrimony of humanity, in as much as they present themselves spontaneously to human minds the world over in a manner that goes beyond any geographical or ethnic linkage. One of their common characteristics is 'numinosity', in as much as they are able to evoke intense manifestations of ecstatic awe and deep fascination when they appear to the consciousness. Jung writes that there are as many archetypes as there are typical life situations. By this expression, he meant the marginal situations that follow the borders of rational understanding. On this subject, Jung writes:

> The contents of the personal unconscious are chiefly the *feeling-toned* complexes, as they are called; they constitute the personal and private side of psychic life. The contents of the collective unconscious, on the other hand, are known as *archetypes*.
>
> (Jung *CW* 9, part 1: para. 4)

Like the *feeling-toned* complexes, archetypes manifest themselves as personalities who act in dreams and fantasies:

> Like the personalities, these archetypes are true and genuine symbols that cannot be exhaustively interpreted, either as signs or as allegories. They are genuine symbols precisely because they are ambiguous, full of half-glimpsed meanings, and in the last resort inexhaustible. . . . The discriminating intellect naturally keeps on trying to establish their singleness of meaning and thus misses the essential point; for what we can above all establish as the one thing consistent with their nature is their *manifold meaning*, their almost limitless wealth of reference which makes any unilateral formulation impossible. . . . As the archetypes, like all numinous contents, are relatively autonomous, they cannot be integrated simply by rational means but require a dialectical procedure, a real coming to terms with them, often conducted by the patient in dialogue form, so that, without knowing it, he puts into effect the alchemical definition of *meditatio*: an inner colloquy with one's good angel.
>
> (Jung *CW* 9, part 1: para. 80, 85)

Because they are relatively autonomous, archetypes can emerge and manifest their presence in dreams, in the dramatic play related to them, in memories, and in the representation of everyday life. The appearance of archetypes is connected with the emergence of a great charge of energy related to the archetype, which marks the passage from linear, historical time into the cyclic and sacred time of the archetypes themselves. Eliade writes:

> Nevertheless, it has been possible to show a continuity between the oneiric and the mythological universes, just as there is a homology between myth-ological Figures and Events and the personages and happenings in dreams. It has been shown that the categories of space and time become modified in dreams, in a way which to some degree resembles the abolition of Time and

Space in myths. Moreover, it has been found that dreams and other processes in the unconscious may present, as it were, a 'religious aura'; not only are their structures comparable to those of mythology, but the experience of living through certain contents of the unconscious is, as the depth-psychologists see it, homologous with the experience of the sacred. . . . The 'religious aura' surrounding certain contents of the unconscious does not surprise the historian of religions: he knows that religious experience engages the whole of man, and therefore stirs the depths of his being. This is not to say that religion can be reduced to its irrational components, but simply that one recognises the religious experience for what it is – an experience of existence in its totality, which reveals to a man his own mode of being in the World.

(Eliade 1967: 16–17)

In psychodrama something happens that is similar to an *epistrophe*. According to Hillman, *epistrophe* starts out from a real-life experience and returns to the archetypal image that underlies that experience. This phenomenon, which appears in real life and in 'role play', is led back to its underlying archetypal and imaginal grounding. Psychodrama seeks to create an 'iconic' or imaginal expression by representing the events of lives that have been lived through. A person starts from everyday life or from memories of it and goes back into imaginal space. Through the performance and the iconic image, a person rises up from his or her role to the archetype that goes along with the role or image. Hillman elaborates on the ways in which archetypal themes influence our consciousness and our ways of being. He speaks of *epistrophe* – reversion or return that consists in leading phenomena back to their imaginal grounding. 'Reversion is a bridge, too, a method which connects an event to its image, a psychic process to its myth, a suffering of the soul to the imaginal mystery expressed therein' (Hillman 1979: 4). *Epistrophe* implies a return to a multiplicity of possibilities and resemblances among images that cannot be explained in any systematic, all-encompassing way.

In this way, a person enters the time of the soul, where 'laws of logic, values, good, evil, and morals are not worth anything. Here there is no conception of time.' The soul that leads a person into a world of the eternal present, a world without history, replaces the ego that historicizes. As in Greek drama, questions about a person's everyday life transform themselves into questions about his or her human destiny. When the actor takes off the mask of the role he has played, he remains alone to question the empty mask, the emblem of the world beyond the tomb and of the gods. Erich Neumann describes the consciousness in its questioning in this way:

If our consciousness, with epistemological resignation, is constrained to regard the question of the beginning as unanswerable and therefore unscientific, it may be right; but the psyche, which can neither be taught nor led astray by the self-criticism of the conscious mind, always poses this question afresh as one that is essential to it. . . . The statement of identity and the logic of consciousness erected on it have no value for the psyche and the unconscious.

The psyche blends, as does the dream; it spins and weaves together, combining each with each.

(Neumann 1993: 7–8)

The psyche tries and always keeps on trying to give multiple, inexhaustible, and allusive answers in the language of images and of myths.

SYMBOL AND ARCHETYPAL IMAGE AS GATEWAY BETWEEN LINEAR HISTORICAL TIME AND CYCLICAL TIME

To repeat, archetypes do represent a person's sort of in-born disposition to produce symbols. These symbols manifest themselves in the shape of images that are able to fascinate the consciousness thoroughly. Jung writes in *Symbols of Transformation*:

> The changes that may befall a man are not infinitely variable; they are variations of certain typical occurrences which are limited in number. When therefore a distressing situation arises, the corresponding archetype will be constellated in the unconscious. Since this archetype is numinous, i.e., possesses a specific energy, it will attract to itself the contents of consciousness – conscious ideas that render it perceptible and hence capable of conscious realization. Its passing over into consciousness is felt as an illumination, a revelation, or a 'saving idea'.
>
> (Jung *CW* 5: para. 450)

In a psychodrama group the archetype can manifest itself through the telling or the playing out of a dream, memory or action from everyday life. What characterizes its emergence is the intensity and also the violence of the emotions that might accompany the archetype's irruption into consciousness. This involves the individual participants but may easily involve the group deeply too, against whom the archetype may resonate intensely. In an almost choral way the participants start to pay attention, involve themselves, feel, and empathize. Jung explains this phenomenon by the fact that archetypes are like behaviour patterns (even though he is referring to a specific patient's experience in the following excerpt).

> This observation is not an isolated case: it was manifestly not a question of inherited ideas, but of an inborn disposition to produce parallel thought-formations, or rather of identical psychic structures common to all men, which I later called the archetypes of the collective unconscious. They correspond to the concept of 'pattern of behaviour' in biology.
>
> The archetype, as a glance at the history of religious phenomena will show, has a characteristically numinous effect, so that the subject is gripped by it as

though by an instinct. What is more, instinct itself can be restrained and even overcome by this power, a fact for which there is no need to advance proofs.

(Jung *CW* 5: para. 224–25)

All this can easily be related to the group level too. This can be easily compared to the irruption of the 'sacred' into profane time. Eliade underlines that any time is open to sacred time. Any time can reveal the absolute, the supernatural, and the prehistoric that emerge unexpectedly in 'incisions' experienced in profane time. The sacred can manifest itself as a lightning opening, an instantaneous interruption in profane time that gives a person a chance to glimpse the 'Great Time' (Eliade 1963: 290).

Eliade maintains that any moment or slice of time can become hierophanic at any moment. If a hierophany is reproduced, this is enough to transfigure and consecrate time because time, once repeated, becomes infinitely repeatable. Archetypes act in the same way in that they keep their identity and their ability to reproduce even though they are infinitely changeable. The meeting of sacred time and profane time – that is, the 'incision', the lightning opening into which sacred time is inserted, as Eliade says, contains the violence that the archetype has when it shows itself to the consciousness. This is the reason why a person has to have a sheltered space where all this is possible for him without making him succumb to the destructive effect that the archetype can have on the consciousness. The passage between one time and another signals extremely critical moments when the *temenos* and the repetition of the ritual serve to protect a person.

As for psychodrama and its relationship with ritual, it is again important here to lead psychodrama back to its historical origins. Dramatization takes it roots in ritual and sacred drama. The events that are represented are those related to the gods and to the myth of the origins. To reiterate Hillman's concept, the gods find their expression in psychodrama just as archetypes, instincts, and impulses do. In fact, Hillman considers psychology a modern myth in so much as mythology can be seen as the psychology of the ancients. In *The Dream and the Underworld*, he considers mythology a collection of tales 'about humans in relation with more-than-human forces'. Things once called gods are now called instincts, or at least are recognized as psychic forces (Hillman 1979: 23).

When time in ritual is counted out and periodically celebrated, this scanned ritual time sets up its own space and draws its own borders. When 'sacred' time is etched into profane time, it gives profane time a reason for being and revitalizes it by linking it with its deep roots. Sacred time does not destroy profane time because it comes forth in a sheltered space.

The ideas of rhythm, repetition and periodicity hark back to lunar and solar hierophanies. In fact, the sun and the moon are connected to a cyclic quality linked to their appearing and disappearing in the sky and to the alternation of phenomena connected with them. These include the day and night, the passing of the seasons, the cyclical renewal of vegetation, the flooding and ebbing of the tides, and so on. Rhythm and repetition also take up considerable space in mythology, folklore and folk tales. The anthropologist Marcel Mauss comments:

> In the legends of sunken churches, castles, towns and monasteries, the curse
> is never a final one: it is renewed from time to time; every year, every seven
> years or every nine years, on the date of the catastrophe, the town rises again,
> the bells ring, the lady of the castle comes out of hiding, the treasures are laid
> open, the guards sleep: but at the time fixed, the spell closes in again and
> everything disappears.
>
> (Mauss and Hubert 1909: 205; Eliade 1963: 392)

The passage from profane to sacred time signals critical moments when everything is possible, as Eliade relates:

> Magic herbs are picked in those critical moments which mark a breaking-
> through from profane to magico-religious time – as, for instance, midnight
> on the feast of St. John. For a few seconds – as with the 'herb of iron' (the
> Rumanian *iarba fiarelor*), and with ferns – popular belief has it that the
> heavens open and magic herbs receive extraordinary powers so that anyone
> picking them at that moment will become invulnerable, invisible and so on.
>
> (Eliade 1963: 391–92)

Thus the idea of cyclical rhythm is linked to the idea of rebirth, renewal, and resurrection in cosmic or vegetal life. Likewise, it may be linked to an interior, individual, and social renewal when it is considered in relation to contact with the unconscious in sacred ritual as well as in analysis or psychodrama.

To repeat, actions, facts and emotions of everyday life often find a place in psychodrama. These often bring to light 'complexes of affective tonality' linked with the personal unconscious. At the same time these daily events ease the way for archetypal contents to come out of the deepest levels of the psyche, the domain of the collective unconscious, and reach into consciousness. For example, a child may have a conflict with her or his mother when the mother makes unreasonable demands and intrudes into the child's personal life. This situation may activate the archetype of the Great Mother who is inescapable and devouring. The child experiences his or her own personal mother and attributes her with threatening characteristics that she may not have to such a degree. However, the energy linked to the archetype will be activated at the same time. This will permit the child, the erstwhile protagonist of daily skirmishes, to transform herself into a mythical heroine who is struggling against the archetypal dragon of chaos and defending the order of the ego's consciousness. Analogously, some rituals relate to the essential activities of human life, which become profane activities only later, such as hunting, fishing, and farming. Rituals make the myth that tells of their divine origins present once more.

> Every time the rite, or any significant action (hunting, for instance) is repeated,
> the archetypal action of the god or ancestor is being repeated, that action which
> took place at the beginning of time, or, in other words, in a mythical time.
>
> (Eliade 1963: 390)

This recognition interrupts profane time, at least temporarily, as sacred time intervenes, sacralizes the everyday and gives it a sense.

In the world of the archetypes, everyday events are made into myth and take on a meaning animated by a mythical-religious conception. Eliade holds that any time is apt to become a sacred time; that is, duration can transform itself into eternity at any time. The imitation of an archetype or the repetition of an archetypal gesture can abolish profane time – duration – and transfigure it into sacred time. From this perspective, every action and every object can acquire the value of a hierophany if it can be linked to its historical root related to a founding tale. This is what happens (as discussed before) in the transformation of space into sacred space. Every action can be linked to a primordial creative act. Thus life assumes the aspect of an uninterrupted repetition of events begun by others through which the eternal history of the world is manifested. A gesture acquires reality, sacredness, and meaning only in as far as it brings one back to a primordial action or refers to it.

To reiterate, psychodrama consists in a continuous moving through time, from the time of the 'here and now' to the time of memories and that of archetypes. Personal memories and contents criss-cross continually, interact with the unconscious of the participants, and so allow personal and group mythologems to be expressed. Alongside the conscious ego that puts into order, historicizes, and tries to recast its memories into its own individual story, the unconscious of the archetypes creates and articulates its own myths. Psychodrama in itself can be considered and experienced as a group dream (where memories, remote recollections, and dreams mix together), and as a passage from a concrete situation to an oneiric dimension. At the same time, psychodrama can be thought of as a chance to experiment and live out one's own dreams in reality with real people.

Archetypes place the 'memory' of the 'space of the soul' where they come from besides the 'historical memory' of one's personal life, which has a very important place in psychodrama. Archetypes relate to the image of a possible consciousness acquired before birth or after death. In *The Origins and History of Consciousness* Neumann relates the 'memory of archetypes' to the 'memory of consciousness':

> In the *Bardo Thödol*, the Tibetan book of the dead, the dead man receives instruction, and the instruction culminates in the doctrine that he shall know himself identical with the 'great white light' that shines beyond life and death. . . . This is what the Jewish midrash means when it ascribes knowledge to the unborn babe in the womb, saying that over its head there burns a light in which it sees all the ends of the world. . . . The mythological theory of foreknowledge also explains the view that all knowing is 'memory'. Man's task in the world is to remember with his conscious mind what was knowledge before the advent of consciousness.
>
> (Neumann 1993: 23–24)

Likewise, the *saddik*, the 'just and perfect one' of Hassidism, the eighteenth-century Jewish mystical movement, is said to 'find' what was lost and bring it back again to men. For Plato the contemplation of ideas existed before birth and knowledge is nothing but the recollection of those ideas.

(Neumann 1993: 24)

In psychodrama two moments interact. In this perspective psychodrama holds out a certain relationship between space and time, between experienced reality and the reality of the archetypes. Thus psychodrama is something akin to Eliade's concept of time as the image of a world that has been made material and endowed with temporal symbolism (Eliade 1991: 34ff.). The lodges of the Algonquin and the Dakota represent not only the world but also the year, which is conceived of as a running across the four cardinal points (the four windows and four doors of the sacred lodge). The image of the circle seen above reappears in the Dakota saying – 'the year is a circle around the world' – and this world is the sacred lodge, an *imago mundi*. In Vedic India, altars like the 'altar of fire' were built with 360 bricks. By building the altar, the world was built again and time, too, was regenerated as it was recreated.

TIME AS IT APPEARS IN GROUP MEMBERS' DREAMS

Historical time and archetypal time interweave continuously in the dreams of the participants. This brings forth a constant composing of the times, epochs, and places expressed through the language of the soul in its ahistorical, Protean, and pregnant tones. In this way the dream can be the object of a backward journey that allows the dreamer to reflect on the dream through the images that appear in it. This going back allows him or her to return to an inner space through amplifying the images whose setting and emotional tone were represented in the dream. This is the *epistrophe* – the name Hillman gives to this resumption of contact with the archetypal grounding in images that the dream derives from. The soul that leads one into the world without history of the eternal present replaces the historicizing ego. In this area the problem of everyday life transforms itself into the problem of destiny, of origin, and of provenance.

As Neumann says of early man, the soul tries with its elusive language to answer vital questions.

> The unconscious knowledge of the background of life and of man's dealing with it is laid down in ritual and myth; these are the answers of what he calls the human soul and the human mind to questions which were very much alive for him, even though no ego consciousness had consciously asked them.
>
> (Neumann 1993: 13)

Here are some examples of images related to time from the dreams of group members. These images will not be followed with an exhaustive interpretation. They can be highlighted best if they speak for themselves. Often, one of the first things that happens in dreams about time is that a clock is lost. Clocks are missing their hands. Clocks disappear. Antique pendulum clocks are rediscovered. Carillons sound the time. Water clocks run backwards or stop entirely. Sundials or positions of the sun indicate the solar hour. All these events enter on stage as points of reference, throwing out often contradictory messages. They tell of a time that is and is not and is free to move in all directions.

> Someone has given me a round watch on a chain that makes me think about the white rabbit's watch in *Alice in Wonderland*. I remember then he was running all the time, always talking in a hurry about promises, but absolutely not understanding where the hell he was going and why. I have the impression that this story is about me and is making fun of me a little. I notice only then that the clock face showed the names of the hours clearly, but there weren't any hands.

> The group leaders lend me a pair of very darkly shaded sunglasses. A voice from out of range invites me to put them on and look at the sun. It is a little past noon and the sun is starting on its slow decline. It comes into my mind that I had become thirty-five last year.

Here the position of the sun seems to be correlated to the person's entrance into what Jung defined as the second half of life, connected with a deep value shift. The analytical work done in the group seemed to bring this out.

> It seems like night almost, but at the same time there's still some sun, even if it makes very little light. I enter a little woods full of briars and trees with dry, contorted branches. I notice that there are chained angels among the branches. I feel obliged to free them.

Here in a twilight of the consciousness that is neither night nor day but an 'intermediate temporal space', soulful and ethereal contents emerge. There are intuitions and thoughts that fly up, imprisoned by an earthly dimension rooted in the ground. The dryness of the branches, their contorted look, and the chains of the angels may call to mind a conflict or difficulty in conciliating the two opposing elements – air and earth. The woman dreamer experienced these elements as a conflict between her creative aspirations that have found no outlet (that can neither move nor fly freely) and her everyday life that cannot become green and put down seeds again as long as it is represented by the prison of the angels.

In the dream dimension, time can run freely in all directions. Past and present can coexist. Time can slip back and forth, and figures and characters from one's own past personal history can show up again, imposing their present reality once again even though they have been forgotten for years, as in the following dream.

> I find myself with some members of the group in a house with a garden. Maybe it is an old *trattoria* in the hills. We've planned to have something to eat

together, but I notice that the house has a run-down, abandoned look. In the garden the benches and the tables are broken and crumbling. Green mould and spider webs are everywhere. Some of the trees are wasted away. Others have fruits that are too small and green on their branches. There is rotten fruit on the ground. Uncultivated and dry grass covers whatever rare flower of the field there is. I see A. come toward me – one of my ex-boyfriends and one of my first teenage loves. I notice he has aged very much and I have the impression that he notices that I too have the same signs of old age. Both of us seem to have an age much older than we have in reality. He talks to me about a thread we have to find in the grass. I then observe the spider webs that are everywhere. I find them beautiful and notice that they hold drops of iridescent dew. Not too far from me A., who seems to have become a teenager again, is designing five-pointed stars inside of circles on the ground with a stick.

In her associations, the dreamer recognizes her own and A.'s premature old age as the ageing and the stiffening of her ability to engage in relationships. She realizes that this is something she had to do again within the psychodrama group that she had just entered at the time of the dream. She contrasted this with the freshness and spontaneity of her teenage love. This contrast is played out against the backdrop of the fruits of the plants – those rotten on the ground and those still unripe and too small on the tree. She was having trouble finding something to eat. She felt that when she was looking for the thread, she was fatiguingly searching for continuity in her story. This would be the plot line that would connect and harmonize the events and characters in her life. She saw the iridescent drops of dew on the spider webs as her hope that her feelings would be born again. She contrasted the colour and feeling to the grey of her everyday life, which she was then experiencing as very burdensome and deadening. She believed her hope to be reconfirmed in the image of the *Animus* of her boyfriend, who had become younger, as well as in the design of the five-pointed star, which she associated both with tarot cards – a current interest of hers – and with a map of the stars.

The search for roots often comes out in groups. These may be understood both as a person's generational roots and as the roots of existence itself. This is something that was illustrated in the dream above by the search for the thread, which served as the point of connection between personal history, group history and the history of origins – the origins of individuals and of the world. When it happens that analytical work in psychodrama stimulates the participants' dreams, the dreams often express multiple familial images including intergenerational lines – grandparents, mothers, fathers, sisters, children, and so on. They appear in the context of the group and take on the same worth as archetypal figures. These generations are linked to the achievements, projections, and expectations related to each participant's own individualized journey and destiny. The image of successive generational lines seems to express the need for continuity between the person himself, his own matrix, and his descendants.

I arrive in the group and I find my parents and my grandmother (by now dead for many years) seated along with the other group members. I then notice that my son is there too. At first I am confused, but then I experience a feeling of relief and satisfaction because the group might be the only way to communicate some things about myself to my family and to try to make them understand those things. Maybe in this context I might manage to understand more of what they are asking me.

At times, instead, the therapists themselves are represented in dreams as taking part in a generational line. Mothers, fathers, children, aunts, and uncles can take on their own identities as images that enable the participants to project welcoming, authoritarian, weak, creative, rational or devouring qualities on to the therapists.

We find ourselves with the psychodrama group in a house with a dangerous balcony, from which we have to lower ourselves into the street by a rope. With us there are my parents, some of my relatives, and relatives of other members of the group. I'm a bit confused about how to lower myself down even if the floor is not very high. Then I notice that W.'s daughter and M.'s little boy are with us. [W. and M. are the group leaders.] Playing agilely and coolly, and they skip over the railing, the first ones to lower themselves down the rope. One by one the entire group follows them and even I find the courage to lower myself down.

At other times, the simultaneous flowing backwards and forwards of time is expressed by the simultaneous presence of figures and images belonging to various historical epochs, as in these two dreams.

Some new participants have entered the group. They are characters from the sixteen hundreds . . .

In a medieval setting I go into the church in what seems to me to be a Benedictine monastery. Inside I see M. [the leader] who is playing the organ in clothes from the period. A little bit farther away I see W. [the woman leader] standing up wrapped like an Egyptian mummy. She is giving oracular answers while falling into a kind of trance. I know that she is living through my anorexia and that she is talking to me about it.

(The second dream will be treated in more detail in the section on initiation disease.)
   The following dream can be related to irruption of the time of the soul into profane time (as treated in the preceding chapter) – i.e. the irruption of the world of the archetypes into the everyday world or, in Hillman's terms, the irruption of Hades on to the earth.

When I leave the psychodrama group, I find myself walking alone at night along the porticoes of a square piazza. The lighting is very dim. I see an old man coming toward me holding a little girl's hand. The old man has something threatening about him and I have the feeling that the little girl is in danger. I feel attracted and afraid at the same time. I notice that the little girl is entirely covered with masks, which prevent me even from seeing her face. When she brushes by, passing close to me, the masks fall down suddenly and I notice that they had been covering a void. I feel the presence of the old man, his back turned from me. I feel a very cold feeling.

This dream expresses the protagonist's fear and fascination at facing the world of archetypes a few sessions after she joined the group. Here the masks represent time understood as the roles and functions that are taken up in life every day. Disquietingly, what emerges beyond that is the dimension of emptiness as absence of time. On the one hand, emptiness can be experienced as a loss of meaning. On the other hand, it can set itself up as a possible container of archetypal images. (This dream will be discussed further in the section on transvestitism.)

This is the sense by which Hillman describes the emptiness that is characterized by the absence of the elements of time and meaning. He compares this absence to Hades, the god of the underworld. In fact, emptiness takes us back to death, the very idea of which can take the meaning out of everyday life (if we understand it as something characterized by time, action, and contingency). However, death can also endow life with the depth and wealth of the soul, which is something experienced as a fascinating and unfathomable mystery. Hillman describes Hades as the void, negation. He is a divinity who is never represented. He has neither temples nor altars. If he is portrayed, he has his back turned. If sacrifices are offered to him, the devotees do it with their backs turned. His impact on the world is experienced as a violation, as a lightning-like irruption connected to the rape of Persephone. It is therefore comparable to the irruption of the world of the archetypes into the world of everyday life and to the laceration that sacred time produces in profane time, as Hillman relates:

> Hades' name was rarely used. At times he was referred to as 'the unseen one', more often as Pluto ('wealth', 'riches') or as Trophonios ('nourishing') . . . All this 'negative' evidence does coalesce to form a definite image of a void, an interiority or depth that is unknown but nameable, there and felt even if not seen. Hades is not an absence, but a hidden presence – even an invisible fullness.
>
> (Hillman 1979: 28)

Hades is hence the god who takes away from the dimension of time and negates its meaning.

This last dream to be treated was brought in by a participant who was working out her separation from the group in order to follow her own journey of individuation after several years of psychodrama and individual analysis.

> I start off walking uphill on a long journey. When I reach my goal, I find myself before a stone slab with *sacerdote in eternis* ['a priest for eternity'] written on

it. Next to it, there is an empty cast of a hand. I place my hand in it and notice that it fits exactly.

In their imaginations the group members later associated the empty cast with an image of empty spaces inside the mountain she was walking up – spaces that reproduce outer reality.

These dreams have had their own space and their own time. The stage has been set for other dreams – the dreams related in the following sections – that are to play a role in the initiation and transformation of their dreamers.

Part II

The constellation of the archetype as transformation

Chapter 4

Introduction: the constellation of initiation symbols in the group's dreams

A person's entrance into a psychodrama group is often marked by a sort of initiatory entrance through a 'narrow door'. Emotions, tears, and a heightened potential for empathy sanction his or her emotional entrance into the group. For psychodrama, entering through the 'narrow door' means that a participant brings some deeply meaningful piece of himself and of his life history to the group. He may feel as if he is giving himself or his dreams 'to the group to feed on' and is letting himself be chewed or ripped up into pieces in the hope of being put together again at a higher level of consciousness.

Entering through this 'bottleneck' is a very touchy phase for a person seeking access to the group. It marks the moment when his or her motives for going through with the experience are tested. In fact, this is the time when he or she may want to get away very intensely. If the participant's motives for this inner search are not deep enough, he or she will start to take flight and abandon the group. However, what happens most of the time is that the affective and protective atmosphere of the group – the *temenos* that has been created in the meantime – is able to support the new participant through the difficult transformative passage. He or she will be encouraged and accepted to regress. As in individual analysis, he will feel that he is able to go through his own 'dismemberment', his recomposition, and his possible resulting regeneration.

The web of themes that are spun out of the dreams, the scenes enacted, and the upheaval in the group often give rise to the same symbolism that can be found in processes of initiation. In fact, the same symbols appear in initiation rituals and function in the same way to link the time of the soul to the historical time of the here and now, the time when the ritual is celebrated. In effect, initiatory symbols appear in the group members' dreams and help develop a kind of individuation of the group as a whole and of its individual members.

What takes place may be said to be what Erich Neumann defines as 'centroversion', an evolutionary phase in the maturation of the ego consciousness. This is a kind of return to oneself and a recognition of one's own ability to reflect and penetrate. In this way a person marks the difference between himself or herself and the obscure and chaotic world of the unconscious (that introversion takes him to). He also distinguishes himself from the anonymity of the collective consciousness (in which an extroverted attitude could get lost). Hence centroversion reasserts the unity of the ego that expresses itself in the individuative path – that is, in the bringing out of a person's human potential and unique and unrepeatable relations. This is something that is opposed to an excess of extroversion, where the subject loses himself in the world. It is also opposed to an excess of introversion, where an individual can be submerged in the strength of the archetypes. Neumann writes:

> The third type of hero does not seek to change the world through his struggle with inside or outside, but to transform the personality. Self-transformation is his true aim, and the liberating effect this has upon the world is only secondary.
>
> (Neumann 1993: 220)

A person starts out by becoming aware of his own 'centre'. He comes to recognize this stable point as something that enables him to confront the loss involved with a sense of an identification with the collective consciousness that is devoid of any inner content. At the same time, a person builds up the strength to resist the dangerous fascination of the world of the unconscious, which may attempt to lower his level of consciousness and work to disintegrate his personality. Neumann further states:

> Centroversion, by building up the conscious ego and by strengthening the personality, tries to protect them and to counteract the danger of disintegration. In this sense, the growth of individuality and its development are mankind's answer to the 'perils of the soul' that threaten from within, and to the 'perils of the world' that threaten from without . . . Stability and indestructibility, the true goals of centroversion, have their mythological prototype in the conquest of death, in man's defenses against its power, for death is the primordial symbol of the decay and dissolution of the personality.
>
> (Neumann 1993: 221)

Hence one can say that centroversion expresses a person's desire and inclination to test himself or herself out as a permanent, indestructible being and to search out something from within that would bring out this potential. The myth of Osiris – his dismemberment, recomposition and the ascent to heaven – is a symbol of such a transformation.

The shaman is another emblem of this process. A shaman rises into the heavens on a magic rope, returns to the earth in pieces, and gets put together magically. His dismemberment occurs at the height of the ecstatic state when heaven has been reached, and the magic recomposition occurs afterwards. The shaman is priest, healer, mystic, magician, seer, and prophet. He or she gathers all these characteristics in himself, but they appear in different measures in different cultures. As is known, the shamanic calling is often manifested through illnesses, ecstasies, visions, or warning dreams, which appear as personal messages.

Various authors – such as Vladimir Propp, Marie-Louise von Franz, and Stith Thompson – have revealed how the same initiatory path is often the very theme that connects the wanderings of the heroes in various fables that can be classified and defined as 'fairy tales' (Propp 1946; von Franz 1990, 1996; Thompson 1946). In these the mythic hero or the shaman destined for a unique future is mirrored in the protagonist. In folk stories this protagonist is often a little girl or boy who may be a prince or a poorer child and who seems to be an initiate. A dream, a vision, or an unusual or unforeseen event – or sometimes an enigmatic or dramatic event – may mark a sharp turning point in the protagonist's life. What occurs here is something like the appearance of a shamanic calling. In the fairy tale and the tale of the shamanic calling, there are often themes that are linked to entering the world of the spirits or of the dead. Both the shaman and the fairy tale hero finish their adventure and re-enter the earthly everyday world enriched by their experiences. However, they face different fates.

The shaman, a person devoted to religion, first goes on an initiatory journey, then usually abandons his or her 'lay' state, distances himself or herself from worldly life, and continues to maintain communication with 'the world of the spirits'. He draws benefits from this world for himself and for his tribe or for the people he is linked with. These benefits include the ability to heal, to draw lots, to predict the future, and to celebrate rituals. The fairy tale hero, however, returns to the world and to his human destiny after he has acquired the treasure, the kingdom, or the princess. What has happened here is also an initiation, but it is more similar to the initiation to puberty that marks the giving up of childhood life and the entrance into adult society (to make an ethnologic parallel).

The 'initiation' in psychodrama is most similar to initiation into adulthood. The protagonist acquires a more mature awareness of himself. He or she returns to the world more aware of his or her acts and thoughts and more responsible for them. This often corresponds to an abandonment of childhood behaviour patterns and actions in which everything seems to 'happen' without any sense of responsibility, or everything is projected on to the external world.

The fairy tale hero's journey and wanderings can often be associated with initiation into secret societies that involve a double, both earthly and spiritual path. Something similar happens when analytical work requires something deeper from a person than the mere resolution of some of his or her symptoms or personal problems. In other words, what happens is that the quest in individual or group analysis or the desire to become a therapist is directed towards an inexhaustible path of research where individual or group analysis marks only the beginning.

Both the shaman's and the fairy tale hero's metaphoric initiations require tests of courage and transformations. They include contact with sacred phenomena, hierophanies, and origin myths (the creation of the cosmos from chaos). In fact, shamanic initiations are openly sacred processes. In fairy tales initiation appears in a more veiled way in the form of contact with the world of magic and the supernatural. There are some legends, such as those of the grail, that share features both of myths and fairy tales. In these, the contact with the sacred is expressed more explicitly through mystical-like elements.

The last feature that shamanic initiation and the fairy tale hero or heroine's adventures have in common is that they both involve intense and, for the most part, incommunicable experiences. Both openly present characteristics of death and rebirth linked to regeneration. There is often an absorption into oneself or a gesture connected to spiritual growth. Often the shaman or hero becomes aware of 'secrets' that have initiatory characteristics. There are often typical themes, such as the meeting of the would-be shaman or the fairy tale hero with various figures linked to the world of the gods or of the dead – the woman of the waters, the lord of the underworld, or the animal helper. These figures play the role of guides. The places appearing in these tales are often remote universes – the centre of the world, a mountain peak, a cosmic tree, the sky above the clouds, or the forest that lets no light in. Often the hero is helped out of his troubles by acquiring magic gifts – the comb that turns into a forest, the helmet that makes him disappear, the invincible sword, the lamp of Aladdin, the magic doll of Vassilissa, the flute with supernatural powers, or the magic carpet. In the end, the hero manages to get the treasure or free the prisoner. The following sections will illustrate how clearly these same themes appear in dreams about psychodrama groups.

In each chapter to follow I set up a theme, discuss how it appears in myth, legend and/or shamanic practice, and present dreams that are variations on each theme. I will be constantly juxtaposing seemingly heterogeneous material – for example, an ancient Egyptian funeral practice and a dream narrated by a group participant. These seeming shifts in focus may seem confusing at first. They are meant neither to be the last word in archaeology nor in therapeutic technique. However, this process of juxtaposition, I hope, will serve to illustrate just how thoroughly initiation symbols appear in the dreams of psychodrama group members and how much we, as people living in so-called modern times, can learn from experiences and peoples seemingly remote from us in time and space.

Chapter 5

The magic tree or *axis mundi*: the ascent

The shaman's ascent into heaven and descent into the underworld play a central role in various rituals where the shaman makes contact with the world of the spirits. This world is often linked to the world's centre, where the shaman draws off his or her magic powers. A central, cosmic axis, aptly defined as the *axis mundi*, connects the earth, heaven and the underworld according to a variety of religious visions, including very primitive ones. The *axis mundi* allows the different dimensions to contact each other and enables 'chosen spirits' such as shamans and mystics to move through the various planes of existence.

The cosmic axis often takes on the form of a tree located at the centre of the earth that acts as the 'umbilical cord of the world'. This happens in more elaborate symbolic representations, like those in central and northern Asia. Norse mythology speaks of Ygdrasil, the world ash tree that Odin attached his horse Sleipnir to. Siberian shamanism pictures the ascent as climbing up a birch tree that has rung-like notches that transform it into a ladder (Eliade 1963: 285, 1974: 269). Climbing up this ladder, the shaman reaches the ninth or twelfth heaven, where he experiences ecstasy. The tree comes out of a hole in a yurt, a circular hut that has the shape of a sacred diagram with a tree as central axis. The hole in the middle of the yurt allows the spirits to pass. The magic rope and the ladder are varieties of the magic tree. All these images are linked to the existence of a centre through which the *axis mundi* – the tie between heaven and earth – passes. The task of the hero, the shaman, or the initiate is to find this connection.

Psychodrama participants' dreams feature the tree and an array of images connected with it. The tree is a kind of stable high point from which a person can observe others and himself or herself. This is the point where it is possible for a person to keep a distance and, at the same time, to keep a very steady contact with the soil through the tree's roots. This is a way of saying that a person can experience the events of his or her own world of emotions and relations and at the same time be a detached observer of them. Within the ritual-like, regular schedule of group encounters and within the framework of the encounters' precise domain of space, time, and human relationships, each participant may be able to find the steadiness of a tree trunk.

In this way the tree can also represent continuity, the common element that each person is looking for at the roots of his or her own individuative path, which winds around inside the complexity of the group. This is the vantage point from which a person can see how the colours of the emotions change and the seasons of the feelings turn. These changes are marked within the unit of every encounter. From here a person can discover again what these changing feelings mean and how they are related. Branches, trees, and blossoms can be linked to a person's own changeable elements – the transformations in moods over the various seasons of life and at various crucial points of his life history.

The group itself and psychodrama technique reflect and enhance this whole phenomenon and give the individual participant the chance to recognize a continuity in himself or herself linked to the uniqueness of his or her own existence. This takes shape as something that goes beyond the continuously changing perspectives and ways of looking at the world that psychodramatic play fosters in each person as he or she encounters and interacts with the other participants.

The theme of the ascent or climbing of the sacred mountain appears in dreams very frequently and in a variety of ways. Here is a particularly meaningful example:

> I find myself in a field whose borders are lost to normal eyesight. The grass is dry and freshly cut and the land is rather arid. The sun is high in the sky and is beating down really hard. In contrast with the rest of the countryside, there is a gigantic tree, which provides shade and freshness, in the middle of the field. I observe leaves and blossoms on the branches that belong to different seasons and are changing constantly. The gigantic leaves are heart-shaped and look like the *ficus religiosus*. Mid-air roots are hanging from above. I climb towards the top, rest in the shade, and build a tree house among the branches. I have the feeling that I am seeing the world with other eyes.

The dream was enacted in the psychodrama group. The protagonist had the impression that in some way his dream expressed a compensation for his being in the group. In fact, images of wide-open spaces and loneliness flourished. The dreamer made the association that he often felt the desire to stay alone and quiet for a few moments after the group sessions. He did this so that the emotions, feelings, and images that came out of the session could settle and find their place and shape within a network of connections and relationships. The tree – as an *axis mundi* – could represent the ordering principle of all of this, the steady starting point and point of reference. In fact, when he was alone, the dreamer managed to notice the changing of the leaves and flowers in the dream. When he reflected on this, he connected this change to the transformation of the emotions and of their colours while they were being dramatized. Thus, the tree as *axis mundi* here too expressed something common to the iconography of diverse cultures and eras – the trunk as a symbol of perennial life and its branches and trees as symbols of regeneration. The dreamer associated the building of the tree house with the necessity for a transformation linked to 'living among the leaves' – that is, with a closer contact with the vital sap and its manifestations, the branches and the blossoms. From up above in the shade of the leaves, the protagonist found himself observing the dryness there is in too rational a consciousness, which he associated with the aridity of the land and the excessively hot sun.

The *ficus religiosus*'s mid-air roots make it a sacred plant in India. In the first place, it is the tree under which Buddha reached illumination. In the second place, its roots in the heavens are linked to the double, earth and sky connection of the upside-down tree. The roots may allude to people's need to 'root themselves' in a spiritual dimension that is not less than the earthly one. Some authors assume that it is exactly this species of tree that inspired the image of the upside-down tree that the sacred Indian texts, the *Rig-Veda* and the *Upanishad*, speak of (Cook 1974: 18). It is the tree rooted in Brahaman, which represents a manifestation of the sacred in the cosmos starting out from a single transcendent root. The dreamer associated the changing of the seasons that was evident in the leaves and blossoms with his difficulty with facing a new season of life. (He was approaching his fortieth year.)

The following is another instance of climbing and seeing the world through other eyes. A South-American legend tells of a boy who finds himself in a *jatoba* tree that is becoming higher and higher (Gifford 1983: 105ff.). The world begins to get further and further away and the boy loses track of time. He hears the tree spirits talking to the stars and learns their names and stories. When he returns to his village, he becomes famous for everything he has learned. The next dream features another tree where it is possible to hear heavenly voices:

> I am sitting under a big tree. Around me there are other indistinct figures, maybe the group. There is an atmosphere of waiting. A. comes down out of the tree. She is playing with a ball shaped like the world. She looks like a little girl to me and, at the same time, I observe her face, which is very marked by age. I notice that she has a trail of light down her back that follows her spine.

A. was a schizophrenic patient who the dreamer, a psychiatrist, was caring for in his work. Here she seemed to some extent to be an Anima figure linked to the spirit of the tree and perhaps aware of its secrets. When the dreamer played the role of A. in the enactment, he said that he had 'heard the voices of heaven'. When he later made associations about the girl, he said that she presented what in psychiatric terms could be defined as a mystic delirium and that she had always fascinated him immensely. For him, she represented an irreducible patient because she always managed to escape and avoid even the slightest therapeutic approach. He had always felt completely impotent with her as a psychiatrist. Her playing with the ball, her infantile attitudes, and her little baby face with aged lines made him always think about death. The trail of light that marked her spine can lead us to think of what yoga doctrine recognizes as the *axis mundi* within the realm of one's own body. (This is something that the dreamer himself associated it with.) Various texts define it as the 'dorsal tree' and identify it with the spinal column at whose base is Kundalini the serpent. Kundalini represents the vital energy that lies sleeping and that the yogi must awaken through discipline in order for him to reach an awareness of the fullness of existence. This permits him or her to reach a new level of consciousness. In figurative art, the dorsal axis (*axis mundi*) appears juxtaposed with representations of different lotuses, the last of which, the thousand-petalled lotus, represents the state of illumination.

The *axis mundi* is represented in religious practice by the structure of the Buddhist stupa, which symbolizes the central axis that the planes of being radiate from. The figure of Buddha himself is connected with the *bodhi* tree, the *ficus religiosus*. Legend and iconography tell that Buddha's mother, the queen Maya, gave birth to him while she was grasping a tree branch. The dreamer pointed out that the bearer of light was a schizophrenic patient and associated this with his need to break away from his own rational schemes that prevented him from 'going further' on his personal quest.

The following is another dream involving the *axis mundi*. Here a tree sprouts forth suddenly out of nothing. This may make us think that an aspiration for spirituality has appeared.

> I notice that a tree has grown on the roof of my house, which I have just renovated. The moment that I remember that I had not planted it, I climb up there to pull it up from its roots, but I notice that it is very strongly rooted. I then realize that the spontaneous force which it grew out of is a very strong inner strength that rises towards the heights. I realize that this was something I had to reckon with. I finally decide to leave it there.

Legends relate something similar to what happens in this dream. A tree that grows on top of a building or on a mountain peak seems even nearer to the sky. According to a Tartar legend, a white birch tree stands at the summit of an iron mountain. In Mongolia, there are tales of a cosmic, four-sided mountain pyramid, inside which there is a tree that the gods attach their horses to. The protagonist had begun psychodrama group work in an effort to 'restructure himself' and his own professional qualities. However, the dream seemed to show that this work had brought something spontaneous and very tenacious to light – the tree – and that it was something directed upwards.

In the next dream a woman group member tends to be going down and not up:

> There is a ladder in the middle of a room in a crowded theatre. You cannot see where it is going. I just go up the ladder. When I observe things there, I notice that it is obvious that this ladder gives us the chance to go beyond the ceiling towards the sky. While I am beginning to go up, Minister D. [then the Italian Minister of Labour] takes advantage of the moment to fondle my rear end. I then let out a scream, lose my balance, and fall to earth.

After the enactment, the protagonist related that when she played the role of herself, she had the feeling that she was being 'pushed too high'. She was impressed that she had found it hard to make contact again with 'concrete reality'. When she played the role of the Labour Minister, she felt she was a very prosaic character, but that she 'had got down to basics', as was demonstrated by having her bottom fondled. She said that she felt like an authority that had to be reckoned with and confronted if she did not want to tumble down from the ladder.

The enactment of the dream seemed to leave the impression that the ascent into heaven was something premature in view of the inner timing of the dreamer, a very intuitive 26-year-old woman. The dream seemed to be a way that her unconscious was telling her not to escape into the heights. Thus her dream presented her with a libido that may have had to channel its energies into the more concrete problems represented by the Minister of Labour. These kinds of problems were capable of influencing her in degrading or dangerous ways, represented by her being fondled and falling.

As we know, the ladder is a variant of the magic tree in its function as link between heaven and earth. The ladder appears as a recurrent motif in myths and fairy tales, just like the tree taken as the *axis mundi*. Shamans from various Siberian ethnic groups climb up birch trees that have rungs fixed to them to help them climb more agilely. In Biblical tradition Jacob's dream of the shining ladder travelled by angels and leading to heaven is an example of the world axis that has been transformed into a magic ladder. Egyptian tombs contain ladders that the souls of the dead could use to climb up to heaven. The ladder is enchanted and so only those who know magic formulas can use it. The god Set is in charge of this. In some visual art Osiris is pictured as a god who is standing at the top of a ladder in his role as guide of the souls from the earth to the heavens.

The image of a ladder that appears miraculously inside a tree or a mountain is a motif that is sometimes found in fairy tales. In one version of *Jack and the Beanstalk*, the plant that Jack climbs up into the sky is transformed into a ladder. Here, too, the ladder represents the element that connects the earth and every-day world with the other world, the celestial realm of the myths. This realm is represented in fairy tales as the realm of magic to perform, of giants and monsters to fight and of deeds to be done. Sometimes the ladder is substituted by iron claws that the hero can climb up in fairy tale motifs. This image of iron claws is linked with the images of birds and eagles, which often serve to carry people off magically into the celestial realms.

In addition, the theme of the *axis mundi* and the ascent into heaven often appears in the form of a climb up a magic mountain and of a summit to be reached. This same motif is found in numerous dreams, some already treated, and some to follow.

Chapter 6

Hermaphroditism

Initiation rites, especially puberty rites, often include rituals that make the neophyte androgynous in some way. An androgynous person frequently appears as a symbol in dreams to bear witness to the fact that a person may be undergoing a transformational process. Such an image involves the *coincidentia oppositorum* and hence gives the person a chance to unite opposites and to overcome the lacerations inherent in duality. This is a process that is undertaken so that a person can get back to his or her original wholeness.

The dream images of androgynization that appear in psychodramatic group and individual analysis often have to do with the integration of the 'anima' or 'animus', something similar to what is expressed in the alchemical process of transformation and the images related to it. These passages are illuminated very clearly by Jung in his *Psychology of the Transference* and *Mysterium Coniunctionis* (Jung *CW* 16: para. 416, 481, 494, 525, 529, *CW* 14: para. 22). Here Jung devotes a lengthy reflection on the symbolic image of Rebis the hermaphrodite (the being double). Rebis represents the philosopher's stone in that she–he is a union of the sun and the moon, of sulphur and mercury, according to alchemical terminology. On this subject Neumann observes:

> Just as the personality gives up the primacy of its specific sexuality and, by assimilating the anima or animus, regains its original hermaphroditism, so the archetypes lose their unambiguous character in a multiplicity of contradictory meanings.
>
> (Neumann 1993: 413)

This is then the way that a person encounters what Jung defines as a 'unifying symbol' or 'transcendent function'. This is produced by a particular situation where the dominating factor is not the hegemony of unconscious creativity, as happens when archetypal images appear spontaneously. What dominates instead is the attitude of the ego towards the unconscious – that is, the strength of the ego.

Psychodrama participants can rediscover their hermaphroditism as a way of getting back in touch with their own cross-sexual potential. This is something that role playing can bring out into the open. It is a way for a person to reunite the opposites of his or her own conflicts by giving both extremes the chance to appear. The image of hermaphroditism can free a participant to rediscover his or her own contradictions, which are expressed in the masculine–feminine dichotomy, when he or she gives voice to them through the group. In role playing, there are rapid passages and exchanges and the dynamics between the sexes are often quickly unmasked. When the participants choose roles and characters, they enable themselves to live and experiment with the other sex as something of their own that is expressed in a variety of moods. In this way personal feelings and emotions may bloom that are connected to the roles that are played. These are the feelings that everyday life does not allow to come forth without having a person pay a price that is at times very costly to society, to his or her own world of relationships, or – what's more – to himself or herself.

Psychodrama legitimizes all these processes through its use of play inside a protected area. However, this does not occur through a person's return to an undifferentiated uroboric state that is threatening and absorbing. Rather, it occurs through dramatic play and the rational consciousness's subsequent working out of this play – something that restores an inner equilibrium. Psychodrama draws and guarantees the boundaries of the space marked by role playing, by the measured time of ritual, and by the identities of each individual participant and of the group. A person's consciousness thus has the chance to reflect, to work out, and to reclaim its emotions and feelings without falling into some kind of undifferentiated mass. In this way a kind of free zone is created where participants can play the roles of the opposite sex, where they can recuperate their own lost creative potential. This is something that is sometimes prematurely repressed, but can now be integrated into the person and enrich the consciousness of his or her ego. When this consciousness finds its soundness in this context, it does not feel threatened.

Androgynization processes are integral parts in initiation rites, especially rites of passage from puberty into adulthood. The following dreams of psychodrama group members feature the archetype of the androgynous person as well as the neophyte's process of androgynization in initiation rites.

> I have the feeling that I am feeling different and that there is something in my physical appearance that has changed. I look at myself in the mirror and notice that I have grown a beard.

This dream brings to mind that the cult of a bearded Aphrodite named Aphroditos was well known in Cyprus, as Eliade relates. The dreamer was a 35-year-old woman who was embarking on a career as a psychotherapist. She associated what she saw going on in the mirror – her process of being transformed into a man – with the transformation she was going through and the identification she was feeling at that time with her professional identity, perhaps excessively. A great deal of her libido was absorbed in her profession at that time. Further, she associated her dream with the fact that most psychotherapists sported thick beards that seemed to instil them with a certain aura of authority. This was a phenomenon in Italy and especially in Turin among her circle of acquaintances.

In any case, she chose a woman to play the role of the image reflected in the mirror in the psychodramatic enactment and she was subsequently invited to exchange roles with this other woman. When she played the role of herself, she felt that looking at herself was an important moment for testing herself out. This was something that provoked a strong emotion in her and disquieted her a little. In her associations, she mentioned some of her experiences with her father. She had always felt extremely valued by him for her intellectual talents. However, she recognized a sort of moral duty to respond to his expectations for her to succeed in the world of masculine values, but this was something that was beginning to weigh on her. When she exchanged roles with the image in the mirror, she felt that there was no beard on the mirror image. Instead, the woman who played the role of her was the one who wanted to see the beard on her mirror image as a sign of legitimization. In fact, under all these appearances she recognized the existence of a rampant femininity in herself that could only remain muffled for a short time and that would subsequently emerge.

Aside from this, what came to light was her problem of competing with the masculine world. This was something she was experiencing in the group and in her personal life. In every case men kept claiming to have 'a longer beard'. They kept insisting on having the last word, even about what she should be or think. In spite of all this, she was able to recognize a kind of masculine inner part of herself that had positive features. In the image with hermaphroditic characteristics, she appeared as a symbol of the unification of opposites and completeness. However, her dream led her to reflect on its negative potential – the fact that these masculine traits could cast a shadow on some of her hidden feminine ones. These perhaps were destined to remain unexpressed at that time both on the personal and on the professional level. She felt that there was a profound wealth that was tied in with her feminine side, which – after all – her most authentic individuality was connected to. She confronted these contents in depth in her successive analytical work.

The following dream of a woman treats an analogous theme that touches on an adjustment to the masculine values of individuality and social success, which are also echoed in her aspiration towards a more incisive position within the group.

> I am seated on the toilet in order to defecate. The realization comes to me that if I knew how to push in the right way, a penis would stick out of me.

Here an archaic 'cesspool' vision is associated with an image of will-power and determination in pursuing one's own ends. After the psychodramatic play, the dream expressed something positive: the woman dreamer became aware that she had new creative potential in herself. In fact, she associated giving birth with the feeling of the pushes that had to be regulated and harmonized. These aspects were ones that the dreamer had not been aware of enough. They were able to express and manifest the masculine aspects of her personality. This masculine potential was something that could bring her towards a harmonizing of the opposites and the tensions she felt she was lacerated by, as she mentioned in her associations. Here the issue was that she could allow her masculine potential to emerge with the penis – seen as her determination and ability to achieve her own projects. This masculine potential was present in her, but had never before come to light in such an obvious way. At the same time, the dream led another group member to make an association with the *couvade*. Among some primitive tribes, the men imitated childbirth while their partners were in labour. They played out a sort of pantomime of birth, the *couvade*, and fell prey to genuine birth pains.

The dream, in fact, seemed again to bring up the antithesis of the two opposite sexual traits and the way they might complement each other. The dreamer wondered, 'What is the use of a penis compared to the ability to have a child?' This later led her to reflect on the antagonism between the sexes and to put women's much touted, so-called 'penis envy' into perspective. This was balanced, if not overwhelmed, by a much deeper envy, men's envy of the power to give birth. This is an envy that is much more repressed. It is probably not an accident that it is mentioned much less, according to current values. The *homunculus* (little man) theory was dismissed pathetically soon after it was posited – the theory that the sperm contains a *homunculus* and that the woman is a mere container that allows it to develop. Further, the self-fertilization of egg cells does not go much higher than the level of tadpoles (as science testified at the time of the dream). All this goes to prove that at this point there seems to be an inevitable encounter and an inevitable clash between the sexes, at least on the biological level. Yet psychodrama takes on this issue by offering its participants the chance to exchange roles and experiment with both sexes.

Conversely, feminine sexual characteristics that express processes of androgynization appear in male group members' dreams.

> While I am shaving, I notice I have a hairless clearness in my beard. In the mirror I have the feeling that I am taking on feminine characteristics. I feel something in an eye, maybe an eyelash, that bothers me to some extent. I manage to take it out and have the feeling that I am seeing the world through other eyes, and that I have a different perception of reality. Maybe it is a feminine vision and it involves seeing the world through a woman's eyes.

This next piece of a dream belongs to another dreamer. In it the emergence of much more overtly feminine aspects is linked to a process of assimilation of the internal figure of the anima: 'I have the feeling that outlines of breasts grew out of me.' The other participants associated the curves of breasts that appeared on him with his nutritive characteristics within the group. The dreamer gathered from his own associations that he had then been feeling that he was keeping in the background those aspects of his personality most closely linked with the rational-masculine sort of thought. These had been overly dominant in his life up until that moment. This change fostered the emergence of that part of his potential more linked to intuition and feeling in his relations with others and with reality.

Similar to the figure in this dream, a bearded Zeus with six breasts forming a triangle on his chest was worshipped in Lambrada in Caria (Asia Minor), as Eliade recounts. The associations that the dreamer made took him to the point of realizing that the group and his analytic work was encouraging certain aspects to emerge in him that were connected to his receptivity and empathetic understanding through feelings and intuition. Perhaps all of this was the 'seeing the world through a woman's eyes' that the dream alluded to.

This next dream expresses other aspects of the process of androgynization: 'When I wake up, I have the feeling that a profound change has begun in me. I notice that my penis has become double.' The dreamer made the association that he had the impression that he had had the chance to 'penetrate' into the two worlds of day and night. The first represented the dreamer's usual approach towards reality through his rational consciousness, while the second was associated with his analytical search through psychodrama. The second penis was something that sprouted up like a mushroom during the course of a night and pushed him to penetrate the world of the unconscious. Known in human physiology and anatomy, the 'hypospadia' that this dream calls to mind is an alteration in the morphology of the genital organs and is often connected with genetic anomalies associated with aspects of hermaphroditism.

Eliade refers to the divine aspects of the androgynous person in his *Patterns in Comparative Religion*: 'The true intention of the formula is to express – in biological terms – the coexistence of contraries, of cosmological principles (male and female) within the heart of divinity' (Eliade 1963: 421). The coexistence of opposites is seen as the typical expression of creative power, which figures among the marvellous qualities of the divinity. In India, the most important divine couple of the Indian pantheon, Shiva–Kali, is sometimes represented in the form of one being, Ardhanarisvara.

This next dream seems to refer to aspects of initiatory androgyny:

> I am having sexual relations with O., who I find to be above me. In one swift movement, she cuts my penis off with a 'cutter'. She tells me that this is a baby organ, like baby teeth that fall out. Strangely enough, this thing doesn't upset me, but I have the feeling that this is something positive, a kind of circumcision needed to become an adult. I will be reborn with a permanent character.

In this dream the archetypal image of the hermaphrodite is represented in its double aspect. On the one hand, the female image recalls the archetype of the great uroboric-phallic mother that the image of castration is linked to. On the other hand, the mutilation that was suffered, which seemed to happen in historical time, recalls initiatory sub-incisions – a topic to be taken up later in relation to pubic initiation into adult sexual life. Figures of the great uroboric-phallic mother are common, widespread throughout all of the Mediterranean area, and are related to the earth and fertility.

After the protagonist played the role of himself in the dream, he related that he felt in some way oppressed by the female figure who was playing an erotic, sado-masochistic game with him. However, this game also had all the playful features of seduction and of a joke – something that he participated in with amused complicity and without tragic undertones. All of this had more of the characteristics of a vaudeville farce.

After the protagonist played the role of O., he said that an initial game of submission was necessary for him to lose his temporary, expiring virility and acquire another more long-lasting one. He related that everything was extremely funny and allowed him to get to something serious involving more commitment that was to follow later. In the associations, the dramatic play brought out the fact that in real life the two of them had to prepare a paper together to give at a scholarly conference. This activity was eroticized into mutual sexual interest. O. had the position as head of the hospital ward where he was working as an assistant, and so she was higher than him in rank. For them to cooperate in a mature way, it was therefore necessary to use a playful means beforehand to neutralize the conflicts of power and competition that would have stood in the way of their work's progress.

The writings of Eliade can illuminate the androgynous features related to the initiatory sub-incisions at puberty as passage into adult sexual life. Eliade writes of initiatory sub-incisions practised among some groups of Australian Aborigines whose aim seemed to be to give the neophyte a symbolic female sexual organ. Eliade writes:

> the deeper significance of this rite seems to be the following: One cannot become a sexually adult male before knowing the coexistence of the sexes, androgyny; in other words, one cannot attain a particular and well-defined mode without first knowing the total mode of being.
>
> (Eliade 1969: 112)

We should remember that the group, psychodramatic play, and the circumstances of analysis help the group members regress. So here it is possible for them to resume contact with an infantile world and way of thinking, where sexuality has not yet been defined. This again brings them to the archetype of the androgynous person. However, at the same time, the group members can structure an ego to observe and reflect on this same regression. In relation to this, Neumann, too, maintains that every individual tends to be naturally disposed toward bisexuality, both physical and psychological, and that he or she is addressed by cultural developments that reject the elements of the other sex in his or her unconscious (Neumann 1993: 413). In group and individual therapy, elements of one's original bisexuality find room to express themselves through images and dreams. In this context, they can be integrated into consciousness.

Chapter 7

Transvestitism: ritual dressing and undressing

Transvestitism – ritual and initiatory dressing and undressing – is a theme closely tied in with that of hermaphroditism. The Siberian shaman is an exemplary figure that can serve to illustrate this theme. According to Eliade, he brings both sexes together symbolically. His costume is often decorated with feminine symbols. He acts like a woman and wears women's clothing (Eliade 1969: 117ff.). Such ritualistic bisexuality or asexuality is often considered a sign of spirituality and of traffic with the gods and spirits as well as a source of spiritual power.

Such features are evident in the following dream, in which a female group member sees the male therapist wearing female clothing and vestments in some sort of pagan–Christian setting:

> I find myself in the middle of a great crowd of people who are watching a procession go by. M. is at the centre in the position of the saint's statue. He is dressed as the Madonna, and decorated gorgeously with female jewellery.

In the enactment, the dreamer recognized that the therapist was reputed to carry *mana* (spiritual power) and that he stood out, being 'decorated gorgeously with female jewellery'. When she played the role of the therapist being carried in the procession, she had the feeling that she was 'weighed down' by the jewels that she was wearing, some of which turned out to be false and particularly heavy. She associated these with her own and the group's projections on to the group leader. Nevertheless, she said that the jewels represented a kind of *ex voto* – that is, a vow involving something of her own that she had to sacrifice so that she could receive 'other' regenerative 'values' in exchange. In fact, the procession could be associated with similar pagan feasts. After the dreamer had got over the slightly sacrilegious irony of the setting itself, she went on to acknowledge the effort that it took for a person to take on such a role.

Dionysus, who has been considered the epitome of bisexuality in a god, is another example of a figure in female clothing. He is linked with the myth of dismemberment and ritual recomposition (as will be treated later). In a way, Dionysus can be thought of as the tutelary deity of psychodrama. In earlier times he was depicted as bearded and robust, but later he appears with effeminate characteristics in many images. As Eliade relates further, even Hercules himself – the quintessential manly hero – and his initiates were dressed as women in mysteries celebrated in *Magna Graecia* (the Greek colonies of Southern Italy) performed to promote health, youth, and vitality. There are many symbolic features in transvestitism and these are related to what was previously mentioned in relation to hermaphroditism (Eliade 1969: 111ff.).

The next dream gives an example of a protagonist who puts on female garments himself. In life he had just achieved an ambition that was as prestigious as it was ambiguous. In the dream this achievement is represented by his signing papers for a project.

> After I put my signature under the president's, I got ready to leave the presidential palace. My camel hair overcoat is no longer hanging on the coat rack. Instead, there is an ocelot fur coat that I put on nonchalantly.

His signature under the president's in the dream represents his wished-for recognition, which in turn gives him the power to let himself go and express his originality and daring.

In psychodrama there is continual role exchange. There are the roles that are exchanged at the conductor's bidding in scenes enacted from a participant's own life or dreams. There are also the roles in other participants' scenes that each participant is invited to play. In addition, a participant may appear in his fellow group members' dreams and find himself acting some role in them, whether he likes it or not, and whether these dreams are shared with the group or not. It is important to consider that a group member's physical presence, ways of moving, and experiences are factors that are brought into the group and that they evoke fantasies within the group that may become conscious to varying degrees. A person's encounter with the other or with others highlights his or her own nakedness under the clothes he or she is wearing and so brings out and enhances 'the shadow' – that very thing that the 'persona's' clothing and cross-dressing had functioned to hide. The group and its analytic work drive its participants to their limits and brusquely put each face to face with personal features deemed 'negative' in relation to an ideal that their ego holds up to them as some kind of touchstone. In this way the shadow acts to limit the omnipotence that a person presumes to have. The shadow represents concrete reality's resistant impact on a person who may try to let himself or herself be moulded by desires.

The group itself – or the image that the group projects – is the same thing as the experience of a person's own finiteness and lack of omnipotence. The group represents the resistance put up by reality. On the one hand, all this may threaten the consistency of the ego. On the other hand, it may be the basis for its enrichment and creative expression. If, however, the shadow is taken out and thrown back down into the unconscious, it acts on its own in amazing ways that are often opposed to the ego's values and plans. Instead, the shadow may change into 'a fairy progenitor of equivocation' who is capable of provoking much graver damage

(Romano 1975: 55). Because the shadow is unconscious, it can be projected on to the group members and therapists who function as sorts of movie screens for them. These projections can be represented concretely in terms of images and in dress. In dreams, the projections range over the themes of clothes put on, clothes swapped or stolen, or clothes worn against a person's will.

> At the centre of the circle formed by the psychodrama group, there is a huge pile of used clothes, like those that used to be found once at stands in outdoor markets. I know that these are the clothes worn and discarded by each one of us and that we have the chance to swap them. The group members hurl them in the air wildly, trying clothes on, trying them on again, and looking for what they feel most comfortable with. Somebody puts on clothes of the opposite sex.

This clothes-swapping free-for-all is a good image of the group itself and of what may happen inside it. Like this dream, many initiation rituals and folklore ceremonies lead to some kind of renewal of life through their focus on the themes of the clothes of the opposite sex and transvestitism.

Androgyny has been expressed through cross-dressing in Polynesia, Australia, and among some African tribes, as Eliade reports. He further writes that cross-gender dressing often used to be practised in ancient Greece. Plutarch himself describes certain varieties of this practice from more ancient times. These were connected with the first nights of weddings, which often came after an initiation into puberty. Cross-sexual masquerades were celebrated as initiatory cross-dressing at some Dionysian festivals in Greece and at the festival of Hera on Samos (Eliade 1969: 113). In rituals and folk festivals transvestitism stands to symbolize that people have come out of themselves, that they have transcended their own particular strongly historically bound circumstances, and that they have re-inaugurated their original trans-human and trans-historical states of being. This is exemplified in European carnivals as well as Indian spring festivals and agricultural ceremonies, as Eliade observes. This process fills the need for people to recreate their primal wholeness – that virgin spring of holiness and power – periodically, even if only for an instant. The atmosphere of the preceding 'used clothes' dream shared with the psychodrama group could be associated with this kind of festive renewal, as its woman protagonist conjectured.

Uncomfortable clothes, fatiguing roles, distorted identities, and unnerving projections are items that group members can have 'rethreaded' by their fellows. The group can also bring some 'tight clothes' out of the closet that group members sometimes discover they have actually been wearing all their lives. They may not know to what degree they have chosen these clothes themselves or to what degree others have chosen these clothes for them. In any case, they may find it hard to take them off, which is the topic of the following dream.

> I am travelling on a train that is taking me to the group. I find that I am wearing a pair of jeans with a high belt, even though I don't know whether I had bought

them or not. They are giving me a lot of trouble and they feel tight like a cilice [penitential belt]. I want to change them, but I know I could do it only if I manage to make all the moves I need to while the train is going forward and while I am standing with my feet on top of a ball in the corridor opposite the individual compartments of the railway car.

The group can make its participants wear 'tight clothes'. It can make them notice that the clothes they find themselves wearing more or less consciously are just as uncomfortable. If so, it can likewise point out to its participants how they can get rid of these clothes when they stand in the way of their progress on their individuative paths. This occurs in the following dream, previously cited in relation to psychodramatic space.

I am in a space where there is a lake in the middle. I see my girlfriend in the water. She is swimming but seems to be in trouble. I realize that I'll have to make an effort to bring her to the shore. I then notice that I have a doctor's white smock on and that I have to take it off before I jump into the water.

After the dream was enacted, the white smock turned out to have a double function. On the one hand it was a professional uniform connected with the 'social status' that goes along with a doctor's prestige. On the other hand, it was a diaphragm that protected against germs and the threat of contagion. Within the context of the dream, the white smock was able to be used to protect the protagonist from emotion by keeping him on the dry *terra firma*, but it turned into an encumbrance that had to be taken off so that the girl could be saved in the water. The protagonist experienced the figure of the girl as the world of emotion and sentiment. All in all, only after the protagonist had freed himself from his own costume and professional *habitus* tied in with the image of his persona (in Jungian terms) was he able to save and rehabilitate his anima as guiding figure.

Here is another dream related to the theme of clothes. In it, there are several images that express the dreamer's problem of 'taking herself seriously' and 'making herself be taken seriously' within the group as well as within society and her family.

I walk into a shoe store because I need some comfortable shoes that would enable me to walk a long way. I point out a dark blue pair with a buckle to the saleslady. These look a bit austere, but they seem to be just what I need. When I put them on, I am let down when I realize that my feet are wearing little pink 'little chickadee' shoes decorated with ostrich feathers. This makes me feel very uncomfortable.

The dreamer was a strikingly beautiful woman who was going through some real anxiety over her frustrated desire for recognition on what she termed 'other levels', meaning the intellectual and professional levels that she felt lacking in. In the dream her desire (the comfortable shoes that she could walk a long way in) was unmasked and checked while she was sent back into her usual role as frou-frou woman (the ostrich feathers).

In her individual and psychodrama group work she had been grappling with her disquiet over not recognizing a more significant, substantial and profound identity for herself professionally, culturally, and even humanly. Likewise, she felt that others denied her such an identity. This was the identity she was longing to be recognized for, something besides her already taken-for-granted recognition of herself as a beautiful woman. Nevertheless, she felt fragile and insecure with any aspect of herself that did not relate to her physical beauty, and so she tended to flaunt her beauty in spite of herself. While her beauty allowed her to win approval, it seemingly overshadowed and slowed down her individuative and maturation processes and unsettled her deeply.

After the dramatic enactment of the dream, she reflected that the feeling of self-assuredness that she flaunted at the beginning of the dream soon gave way to shame at being unmasked as the little ostrich feather shoes appeared. She associated the role of the saleslady with the function the group had for her of unmasking her weaknesses, sometimes far too cruelly. Likewise, she also recognized this same feature in herself – her attitude of undervaluing herself that she found she was fighting. In her subsequent group and individual work, she often used the metaphor of the 'ostrich feathers' to help her focus in on some of her moods. Here her persona (in the Jungian sense) had been useful for her in obtaining the social integration that made her happy at times, but it jeopardized her chances of going beyond this. As the dream relates, her persona had been trapping her and turned out to be a garment that might not be able to be exchanged for anything else. Furthermore, such rigid and almost inflexible roles – often tightly linked to image of the persona – may sometimes function to ease a person's superficial adaptation to circumstances, but can easily turn into a prison. Such roles can act like the shirt that Deianira gave Hercules, as legends relate. This was a shirt that turned itself into a trap: it could not be taken off except at the price of life of the wearer. Psychodrama attempts to give its participants the skill to recognize such clothing traps and perhaps to neutralize them, or at least to limit their negative power by learning to unravel them with aplomb.

It is the function of psychodrama to offer people the chance 'to change their clothes often' so that clothes and roles do not stick to the skin inextricably. This enables people to tell the difference between their own nakedness and their clothes. In other words, they can distinguish between their own essence – the ego linked to the Self over the course of the individuative path – and their roles. These are the roles and the more fleeting, changing characteristics that the group and life in society keep on throwing out at people. This is the only way that losing one's clothes, one's role, and the features linked to the persona does not lead to the fragmentation of the ego. When the ego is represented in its nakedness, it is made more stable by being linked with its more profound essence, the Self. All this is expressed in lively images in the following (previously cited) dream:

I find myself on a trip with the psychodrama group on a horse-drawn wagon that has all the features of a circus wagon and of a knick-knack cart. In the middle of it there are old and new clothes of all styles and sizes, used shoes, costumes from melodramas, clown suits, make-up equipment, jewels, and flowered straw hats. I notice I have only my underwear on and at first this creates a certain uneasiness in me, but bit by bit I realize with satisfaction that this will let me put on everything more freely.

In psychodrama group work, participants and conductors closely observe and try to intuit which person has dressed up in disguise and what the disguise is. They want to be able to 'strip the person naked' and 'unmask' him through dramatic play, through having him play a role, or through a dream that indicts the image he has of himself, even against his will. It sometimes happens that a person unmasks himself or herself by recounting a dream, by changing roles in role playing, or by sharing a real-life experience with the group.

At times unmasking gives the person unmasked a sense of relief because he feels that the shadow parts of himself have been revealed, exhibited, elaborated, and accepted by the group – aspects that he would never have had the courage to reveal so freely. At other times, the moment proves not yet to be ripe for working something out and, as a result, shedding light on a person's shadow may provoke embarrassment, tension, and unease. Nevertheless, what is important is that something comes out into the light, that something stirs up the waters and allows a static situation to be broken up, and that something frees up the flow of transformations of consciousness, emotions, and feelings. The images in the following dream illustrate the freeing up of the flow of a person's own emotions and feelings and his ability to express them freely. It was related to the group near the time of the temporary summer break in the group's activity when some members try to take stock of the group's evolution over the year and in some way sum things up.

Several people in the group are showing their underwear. There is freedom in this gesture, but also ostentation. The first one to show her underwear is L., lifting up her skirt while laughing maliciously. G. and N. do the same. The group makes a show of its ovations and comments at every exposure. Even a bit on the sly, I realize that, in fact, all of us are gradually taking all our clothes off and heaping them up in a corner of the room. There are some people who are showing their underwear nonchalantly, and some who aren't. Later we all find ourselves in our underwear. I realized at last that the message of the dream is that the group is off to their conclusion 'in their underwear'.

The dreamer associated the female group members who stripped first and provoked applause with their ability to show their feelings and cry in the group. He called this their 'knowing how to show their panties with cool but without losing face', which he related to their work in the psychodrama group. He pointed out that their gestures were so free yet so exhibitionistic. This led him and the group to reflect on the space a participant could mark out for himself or herself and on the power that could be gained when he or she had the savvy and the skill to show his or her own emotional world. Such a person earned space inside the group, inside the dreams, and inside the emotional experiences of the other participants. This experience coincides with an Italian saying: 'to end up in underpants' or 'canvas pants'. This means to have nothing else to lose and so to have the strength or be 'constrained' to show one's nakedness and everything that goes deeper than appearances.

This theme of nudity appears in many alchemical, religious, and folk traditions. In the *Rosarium Philosophorum*, a book illustrating the phases of the alchemical process that Jung examined for his studies on transference, the king and queen emerge nude from the purifying fountain. Transformation begins with nakedness. Similarly, initiates immerse themselves in baptismal water nude and emerge regenerated. In the *Panavinca Brahamana* and in many other traditions in Vedic India, to shed 'one's own skin' like a snake or to free oneself from an animal hide plays an important role in rituals. This role comes into play from the moment when this shedding begins and means, metaphorically, a person ridding himself or herself of his profane condition, of his or her sins, and of old age in order to enter some kind of superior existence (Eliade 1969: 91). The same theme is taken up again in many folk tales that follow the plot line of the Grimms' *Donkey Hide*, *The Frog Princess*, and *The Swan Girl*. In these the heroine's royal blood or underworld origin alludes to a connection with the Self. She wanders a long time inside an animal hide and then manages to free herself and take sovereignty over the kingdom. In the following (already cited) dream, the infinite multiplicity of clothes and roles is represented through the image of a garment of masks that cover a void:

> When I leave the psychodrama group, I find myself walking alone at night along the porticoes of a square *piazza*. The lighting is very dim. I see an old man coming toward me holding a little girl's hand. The old man has something threatening about him and I have the feeling that the little girl is in danger. I feel attracted and afraid at the same time. I notice that the little girl is entirely covered with masks, which prevent me even from seeing her face. When she brushes by, passing close to me, the masks fall down suddenly and I notice that they had been covering a void. I feel the presence of the old man, his back turned from me. I feel a very cold feeling.

In the dramatic enactment, the woman protagonist chose the female group leader to play the role of the girl clothed in masks. This character deeply unnerved and attracted her at the same time. In the subsequent role exchange she played this part herself. After this enactment, the protagonist reflected that she had the feeling that she herself was the girl in the dream. She associated the masks with the changeablity of roles and expressed feelings – her own and others'. Yet she allowed herself, above all, to give vent to her most disturbing questioning about what is left on the other side of the masks, about whether a person can change her essence by changing her clothes, and, if so, about how she can do this. When the masks clothing the girl fall off, the uncovered void clarifies the dream's disquieting and sometimes anguishing aspects. This is determined by her fear of encountering her own lack of consistence, transitoriness, and relativity to existence itself. Enacting all this had the effect of transforming the fear of emptiness she lived through in the dream into awareness.

As Kerényi reminds us, the empty mask without a wearer is an instrument in the mysteries that became a cult image (Kerényi 1949: 193). It symbolizes the presence of the god itself without the mediation of the human wearer. It is in front of the empty mask placed as cult object in forests, near streams, and near tombs that people were led to question into their own fates marked by time, destiny, and death.

Chapter 8

The sacred meal

The shared preparation and eating of food is a theme that often turns up in dreams brought into groups. The preparation, consumption and digestion of food immediately seem to express many of the participants' expectations symbolically in regard to the group's implicit goals. In other words, there is a mixing of everyone's ingredients, stories, fantasies, characters and dreams. What happens is that this raw material is cooked up and transformed, and the resulting concoction contains everyone's projected expectations for nourishment and regeneration. In any case, the nature of the foods often depends upon the circumstances themselves. Food is the figurative expression of what the participants have brought in from among their emotions, feelings and moods. It is the job of the therapists to bring all of this together and make it palatable as nourishment, as happens in this dream.

> I find myself seated at a table with the other group members at the entrance of the psychodrama group room before the session is to start. A common meal is coming up. The dishes – cooked and raw foods – have been prepared by W. and M. with the help of the others. The therapists are serving the dishes at the table. There are strange foods, which cause a certain squeamishness. There seem to be good quality ingredients, but they seem to have been combined badly. Or, at least, the combinations are weird and unusual.

When the dream was enacted, the protagonist played the role of himself. He then associated the dishes offered to him with some of his moods and the ways they were dealt with in the group, which he felt were inappropriate at the time. This made him feel somewhat 'displaced' from his normal ways of being and representing himself in public. All of this led him to reflect on some of his self-contradictions and work them out. When he exchanged roles and chose to play the role of one of the two therapists (who was also male), he felt that he had the task of making elements coexist that were hard to reconcile even though these elements were his own values.

The ingredients of foods and all kinds of bizarre and arcane recipes, which, nevertheless, were often appropriate to the occasion, came up rather often in the dreams of the psychodrama group. They came up so frequently that it led some group members to suggest that they draft a sort of 'psychodramatic *Artusi*' (the classic Italian cookbook). Here is the first of several examples: 'I invited my parents to dinner and the psychodrama group members are helping me prepare a special dish. It is called Herb Warrior.' The protagonist, a 32-year-old woman, was living through a difficult career switch at the time of the dream. She was leaving a safe, quiet, but monotonous, job as a government office worker in order to dedicate herself entirely to psychotherapy and art therapy, activities which she had previously undertaken only part time. She had not yet told her parents about her decision even though the deadline for the change was coming up fairly soon. She could not be forced to change her mind, but was still afraid of their negative reaction. Basically, her decision had been brought to maturity in the group. She asked the group members to work with her in preparing the dish through which she could finally present her parents her decisive energy and courage – the warrior – and at the same time the sincerity of her plans – the herbs. These were the associations that she shared with the group after she enacted the scene.

The following dream illustrates that preparing the food is just as important as eating it.

> The psychodrama group is preparing a meal. Everyone is sitting in a circle. At its centre there is a big cauldron boiling over a wood fire. Every once in a while someone gets up, goes near the pot, stirs, checks how cooked the food is, smells, tastes, and adds some ingredient. As it is being stirred, I notice that there is a shoe cooking in the cauldron too. . . . A mayonnaise is being prepared. Everything is there – eggs, lemon, and oil. The ingredients are to be mixed carefully, because otherwise the mayonnaise will break like crazy.

Each of the group members adds his or her own appetizing or disgusting ingredients and spices. The group – the circle, cauldron, container and alchemical vessel – is expected to perform a transformation and render its participants' dreams, fears, and emotions appetizing, digestible, and, above all, nutritious and metabolizable for them. So, it is not surprising that ingredients may be put together poorly (as in the first dream cited) and that this puts the participants' intestinal fortitude to a stiff test. The shoe simmering on a low flame with the other ingredients can be made to fit a person's feet, wrapping them in the real and symbolic matter being processed in the cauldron. It can be made to touch the soil, to be exploited in the everyday world, and not just to remain isolated in symbolic space. The shoe is made out of leather, an organic material that has been transformed, reworked, and made useful, but it cannot be digested. Likewise, everyday life can be just as indigestible if it is not made to come alive through a dialectical relationship and contact with the unconscious and the world of archetypes.

The cauldron, the cooking, the required tending, and the waiting recall the procedures of alchemy and the role of the initiate in them. In addition, the arrangement in a circle and the collective meal preparation can also recall the image of esoteric sect encounters, where the group consumes its own ritual quality and rites of initiation. Hillman relates:

> The alchemists had an operation called *cibation* ('feeding') and one called *imbibition* ('soaking' or 'steeping'), in which the psychic stuff that one was working on required the right food and drink at a certain moment during the opus of soul-making.
>
> (Hillman 1979: 173)

In our case, however, the celebrant is not alone in the alchemical laboratory or paired with a *soror mistica* (mystical sister), but is in a group. Hence the problem comes across under two aspects. There are not only the *daimones* of one person, but also those of the others who share the cooking in the cauldron. This obviously causes a certain amount of distrust to float around. Others could throw ingredients into the pot that a person thought he or she was already free from or had hidden away. These could come floating up to the surface again during the boiling – stuck together, tangled or mixed up with other people's ingredients. It is a sure thing that such a meal is no longer a fancy food banquet.

If the foods are not prepared and transformed carefully enough, it can happen that a mayonnaise could break. Mayonnaise, after all, is a product that requires accurate preparation. It is not only nutritious, but contains an assortment of the components essential for the human constitution – proteins in the eggs, fats in the oil, and vitamins in the lemons. It turns out well when these components mix well and it breaks when they separate out. To prevent this from happening, therapists should carefully supervise the cooking and not hesitate to put some shoes in the potion, which can guarantee a good contact point with the earth and reality at the end of the session. The mandala-like circle of the group members thus maintains the function of containing, protecting, and harmonizing discordant forces.

'Images are the soul's best food', according to a romantic notion that Hillman relates (Hillman 1979: 174). What we eat in our dreams is not food but images. We should therefore pay attention exactly to what people are eating in dreams and where and how and with whom they are eating because these tell us the way that the nutritive process is taking place. Eating in dreams answers a psychic need for images that nourish. Food of any kind represents the very image of nourishment. Everyone gets a different kind of nourishment from dreams. Similarly, each participant is nourished differently from the psychodrama group at varying moments of his or her own personal history and history in the group.

There is a sacrificial atmosphere that transforms eating into a ritual for the psyche, according to Hillman. A dreamer can sometimes have the sensation that he has sacrificed his dreams, that he has lost them through expropriation, or that he has given his own dreams to the group to eat and found them again transformed or distorted when they were enacted. The meal can become a cannibals' feast at some tense moments. Group members may say that they feel devoured or ripped to pieces (a point to be treated in the section on ritual dismemberment). This can also happen to the dreams that are brought into the group. With this risk in mind, it is important for a participant to repossess his or her own subjectivity within the group. This will become an individuative moment for the person that will make him or her aware of the different features and messages in the dream in itself and in the dream in relation to the group. Therefore the dream enactment is a moment of interaction of the ego with the other. Sometimes the dream can be experienced as a sacrificial object that is immolated in the group and the enactment that follows its narration can be disappointing. However, the 'sacrifice' can become fruitful if it enables a person to follow the transformation of the archetypal images that it evokes.

In dreams the souls of the dead may appear at a banquet for the living as a moment of sharing and exchange, as follows:

> I find myself at a table with the components of the psychodrama group. Mingled in with them there are my dead mother, father and brothers. There is a certain sacredness in the sharing of the food.

This dream came after a session in which the protagonist had acted out some difficult moments of her past history that involved the by then dead family members from the dream. In her subsequent reflections, she regretted that she had not been able to untie some knots and settle some conflicts with them before they died. In the dream she was given a second chance and permitted to 'nourish herself' again in her relationship with her inner images of them. As Hillman points out, banquets with the dead are related to Hades, 'the hospitable', who is 'the hidden host at life's banquet'.

As this dream shows, the return to life of deceased relatives in dreams testifies to family influences and expectations that were not achieved by the dreamer's ancestors during their lives. These expectations become part of a kind of family myth instead. These figures make themselves felt at times by giving people the impression that they have some important mission to carry out. In the last analysis they may even represent aspects that the deceased people may not have experienced in their own lives. Besides these figures in dreams, there are the 'pseudo-shadows', as Ernst Bernard terms them – i.e. the shadow (in the Jungian sense) features of parents and ancestors, features that live and relate with each other and with unconscious aspects and autonomous complexes inside the subject him or herself (Bernard 1978: 156). These are the themes that emerged in the reflections following the enactment of the dream.

There is a theme similar to the meal shared with the dead that appears in many Russian folk tales. In this case the sorceress represents an image connected with the underworld. She offers the hero some enchanted food that allows him to pass into the world beyond this one. Symbolically, the food purifies the man from all that is earthly and transforms him into a spiritual, flying, and bodiless creature. The meal of the hero or heroine often plays the critical role in Russian folk tales, as is recounted by Vladimir Propp (well known for his studies on the folk tale's morphology and historical origins). In his research, Propp considers the parallel between the wanderings of the hero of the tale and his initiatory journey. Often the hero finds a little house mounted on a chicken's foot at the edge of a forest. He may find the table set and furnished with food inside the house, or he may find that this little cabin is made from edible and appetizing material – that it is propped up on a pastry or covered by a fritter. This corresponds to the gingerbread house in the more western *Hänsel and Gretel*. A constant characteristic of the sorceress is that she gives the hero something to eat and feeds him.

Likewise, the charmed food that allows the hero to enter the world of the dead is a theme that appears in the Babylonian epic of Gilgamesh (Propp 1985: 110). Visitors to the underworld are offered roasted meats, baked breads, and water poured from goatskins. In ancient Greek mythology Calypso wants Odysseus to nourish himself on ambrosia so that he will have to stay in her power. Similarly, whoever eats the lotus forgets his homeland and stays in the land of the lotus-eaters (Propp 1985: 110). Persephone herself was to belong to Hades after she ate the pomegranate. The folklore motif of the food offered by a sorceress to a hero on his journey to a distant kingdom seems to be based on the magical food given to the dead person on his journey in the world beyond. Propp relates: 'In the Egyptian cult of the dead, food "opens the mouth of the dead". Only after tasting food can the dead person talk' (Propp 1985: 108).

The last course in our treatment of dream material is dessert:

> In the group they are preparing a pie without milk and without yeast. It is being cooked by the light of an artificial lamp. G. and M. [two males – a participant and a conductor] are supervising the cooking. Annoyed, I say that you can't bake a pie like that. A dessert needs milk, yeast, and attention.

This is a dream that a participant brought in shortly after she joined the group. It seemed to express her difficulties in relating to the group itself and to a male rational element which, she thought, took up too much space in the group. G., a long-time group member, presided over the kitchen along with group leader M. She thought that G.'s strong rationality acted as a cover for his affective and emotional side. On more thorough reflection, the problem that was brought forward in the dream seemed to relate to a masculine rationale that belonged to the dreamer herself. This rationale tended not to leave room for her feminine 'milk and yeast' to express themselves and implied that she could 'bake pies' cooking with artificial light. This attitude proved to be projected on several group members and on the group itself, which was basically chided for too much rationality and too little warmth. After this dream the other group members were perhaps a bit defensive in their reflections. In response, other dreams relating to the group emerged a week later which, according to one member, 'transformed the unleavened pie into a St Honoré pastry'.

Chapter 9

Ritual dismemberment

The dismemberment and recomposition of the body is another theme that runs through religion, mythology, folklore, and the dreams and experiences of psychodrama participants. The shaman, for example, is taken apart at the height of his ecstatic state when he has already reached heaven. As discussed previously, he is put together magically again and goes through a mystical resurrection. This same theme appears in Nordic fairy tales of Siberian or Irish origin and in the magic tricks of Indian fakirs and Chinese musicians. The ascent to heaven often occurs by the means of a magic rope that sometimes has knots in it like the rungs on a ladder that make the climb easier. There is also a legend that holds that Buddha climbed up to heaven on a magic rope, came back in pieces, and put himself together again with magic (Eliade 1969: 160ff.). There is another legend, this time from Irish folklore on the Isle of Man, that tells of a magic rope that a magician throws up into a cloud. He makes a rabbit, dog, a lion, other animals, and an apprentice climb up the rope. They are then dismembered. The apprentice falls down to earth and is then put together again. Similarly, the myth of Dionysus includes the theme of his dismemberment and magical rebirth, as discussed in the section on the historical origins of psychodrama. As the god of theatre, Dionysus's mystery cults are at the origin of sacred drama and psychodrama itself.

Dreams of dismemberment, evisceration, and mixing body parts recur with a certain regularity in dreams related to psychodrama groups. When group members speak about themselves, their moods, and their dreams, they often say that they are being 'ripped apart' and 'torn to pieces'. Actually, what is often being ripped apart or torn to pieces in the psychodrama group and individual work is the Jungian persona (Jung *CW* 7: para. 243–53). This includes the image of him or herself that a person shows to the world, the rigid roles that a person is used to playing, or the image of an ideal, stereotypical ego that a person hopes to live up to. The 'ego' that is 'torn to pieces' is something that is strictly identified with the persona, or something that, in any case, has lost its vital and creative interior and therefore has stopped being rich, genuine, and agile. It is something that Donald W. Winnicott terms very clearly as the 'false Self' or 'adapted Self' (Winnicott 1971: 14, 68, 87, 102). This is the issue that groups turn out to be the most ruthless about.

Dismemberment, fragmentation, and the resulting pain are the only things that can lead a person through suffering into greater self-awareness and subsequent re-composition. When a new ego is remade like this, it starts out from a deeper, more authentic inner 'centre' that it stays in contact with in a dialectical relationship. The individuative process goes towards this objective. It can therefore be said that dismemberment, loss of identity, and the resulting suffering together correspond to the alchemical phase called *nigredo*. Jung compared this phase to a deep initial depression, psychologically speaking. This is something that is often met with in the process of analysis, something that clears the ground for the transformation to follow.

The theme of dismemberment is at the core of the issues raised in the following dream related to groups.

> I find myself being transported on a stretcher in a sort of hospital that has very long hallways. There are spacious and large chambers whose doors open on to the hallways. Hospital aides are rushing past me who are transporting stretchers with organs on them that seem like they have just been extracted. There are livers, stomachs, lungs, kidneys, intestines, and hearts. I have the feeling that they are still alive and throbbing, and this repels me thoroughly. I do not know if I have already gone through or if I am about to go through the same kind of operation. However, a sensation of relief comes over me as I feel that I am going towards the end of the hall. Here, someone tells me that the organs are going to be put back in place after their circulation is reactivated. I recognize G. and D. in doctor's smocks at the door.

This dream came after a period of profound apathy and depression in the protagonist when she felt as if she was 'in pieces' and unable to feel any emotions after a disappointment in her love life. When she enacted the dream, she realized that she was completely drained, emptied, and devoid of strength as she entered the hospital, which she associated with the psychodrama group. She associated the organs moving around on the stretchers with intense emotions – emotions that she felt were going around in the group and that she had never managed to put into a context (the heart as sentiment, the liver as rage or courage, etc.) Therefore the group–hospital functioned to bring these emotions to light so that people could observe them and reactivate their circulation. In this instance, the group had set off fantasies about dismemberment, but it had also given her the chance to regain contact with her emotions through suffering. (In fact, the organs were put back into place after their circulation was restored.) G. and D. were two group members who had recently brought their experiences of intense pain into the group – experiences that had shaken her profoundly. Here, they take on the roles of surgeon-therapists.

Another group member dreamed these two dreams, one right after the other, both featuring evisceration:

> I enter a butcher shop to buy meat for lunch. Hanging from hooks on the walls, there are skinned, quartered, and beheaded animals. I am repulsed when I notice that they are still moving and giving signs of life . . .

I have a quartered rabbit in my hand. I am holding it by its feet with the head down. I am in front of the toilet. My little cat is at my feet, who is meowing insistently because she is waiting to eat. I rip out the rabbit's innards for her, but they fall into the toilet bowl. Then I notice that the rabbit is still alive. The group around me is watching the scene in silence.

The second dream was enacted in the psychodrama group. When the dreamer played the role of herself, she felt that she was acting impulsively, as if her very actions were determined by the fact that she was reacting to something. It was something that she felt threatened by even though she could not manage to identify what it was. At the same time, she experienced a deep disgust for what she was doing. When she exchanged roles and played the part of the rabbit, she felt that she was the victim of a painful and useless sacrifice. The innards that were torn out to nourish the cat ended up in the toilet bowl. The cat herself was associated with the protagonist's spirit of independence. With some pain, she recognized the extracted innards as a problem in her own personal history that she had repressed and put aside up until that moment. Namely, she had denied the visceral part of life and her feelings that had been revolving around her desire for motherhood. It then became clear that she had offered the sacrifice under the illusion that she was nourishing her independence (the cat) – a seemingly fictitious independence at that moment in her life. The associations she made with the rabbit – an extremely prolific animal once used for pregnancy tests – led her again to the theme of fertility.

When she reflected on all this after the dramatic play, she associated her dream with a kind of 'voluntary sacrifice' and with her own drastic 'ripping out her guts' in reaction to her family model, which she felt had been imposed upon her in some way. This model featured her mother, the female slave to what she felt was a suffocating biological role.

Her mother, of southern Italian origin, had had many children. When the protagonist was a little girl, she experienced her mother as someone worn out and destroyed by the weight of her family who kept on fantasizing about never getting married. Although the protagonist acknowledged that there was something unavoidable in what had happened, she said she had a painful feeling of deep mourning, something she had not recognized nor yet wept over before. For a long time afterwards, this became the focus of her individual and group analysis, where this issue could be worked out. Eventually, a white female cat appeared in her dreams. It fascinated her and led her to unexplored parts of her house. When this happened, the dreamer recalled her earlier dreams. The cat now seemed almost purified by the whiteness of her fur. She associated the cat with her curiosity, with her urge to seek things out, and with her spirit of independence. All these now seemed to be freed of the deep hunger that went along with the call for sacrifice.

The following dream expresses the same set of issues around the temporary rejection of the feminine and the body in its aspects of sexuality and fertility. Here the violence of the images seems to stem from unconscious contents that have been ignored too long. The protagonist was a 37-year-old woman who had focused very much on making it professionally in her life and had met with some degree of success. However, her personal and emotional life had been put aside, most of all most recently, to benefit other more intellectual ambitions.

> I find myself in the city of B. with a man who may be E. [an ex-boyfriend of the dreamer in her youth]. He tells me that we have to see some important ruins in an old half-gutted-out church. It is called the church of 'Cristo-foro' [a play on words in Italian – *Christ-hole/Christo-pher*] and I am amazed that I had been in B. for so many years and I had never seen it before. I find myself in front of something. It is both a 'statue-painting' and a living being with neither arms, nor legs, nor a head. I realize that it is alive and it is moving. I feel a sharp pang in my stomach and intestines.

This dream was the expression of the re-emergence of her long-forgotten feminine side. When she acted out the dream playing the role of herself, the protagonist rediscovered the feeling of abandoning herself trustfully and of letting herself be led. She had the impression that, all by herself, she would never have found that place. She recognized that her attitude was passive and entirely feminine. That made her think about the fact that she rarely let herself have something like this in her own life. She associated this with a relationship she was having and with the psychodrama group. In both situations, she gradually felt the same feeling emerge even though it came across in a painful and contradictory way. All in all, she now felt she could trust. When she played the role of her male companion – an animus figure – she felt that she trusted his guidance and their goal had something to do with their relationship. When she played the role of the 'statue-painting', she decoded a personal message about the flesh, menstruation, and the womb as ability to procreate. When she played this role, however, she felt that she was detached from the ground and from reality. She could only be a symbol. Her further associations made her realize that the image of the 'statue-painting' highlighted the middle of the body. She associated this with the abdomen, which she felt as the emotional side related to the functioning of the feelings. On the other hand, she thought that the arms and legs were linked with the function of the senses and with going around in the world. She took up the issue of the name of the church of *Cristo-foro*, underlining the word *foro* (a drilled hole). She linked this to her feeling she had to rediscover a hole from which something important should re-emerge.

The recomposition of the corpse is a theme that goes along with that of dismemberment. This evokes the myth of Osiris (Horus), both similar and dissimilar to that of the shamans treated previously. In the case of the shamans, their bodies are cut apart and put together again while they are still alive. In the case of Osiris, the transformation must pass through the phase when the body is dead. For this reason, resurrection represents something that comes after physical death and is connected with the cyclical renewal of vegetation. Neumann considers the corpse's burial and entombment as a kind of ritual meant to perpetuate fertility connected with an eternal potential for rebirth and resurrection. The eternity and fertility of the spirit are parallel in ritual to the eternity and fertility of nature. This is manifest in the cult of Osiris's permanently mummified phallus, which is reserved with its seeds near the corpses until the feast of the resurrection (Neumann 1993: 249).

Dismemberment, laceration, sowing and harvesting mean – as Neumann relates – that the personality is annihilated and that the living unity is destroyed in order to bring about regeneration. What follows is a dream in which a mummification ritual like that performed by the priests of Osiris caused a deep spiritual transformation to come over the people who were celebrating it.

> I find myself on the half-basement level of an institute of Pathological Anatomy along with other group members. We have on the rubber gloves and aprons that are usually used in autopsies. There is a cadaver hanging from its feet from the ceiling in the centre of the room. Our task is to stitch the inner parts together again and to go on to a kind of mummification as we keep on pouring some liquids inside the body. However, some slimy whitish liquid is dripping from the body and we are all getting soiled with it. I am aware that I have to master the deep feeling of disgust that I have. When the job is over, I go up a short flight of stairs and find myself in a 'purification room' where they get rid of the soiled clothes. I wash myself carefully. In the room, there are wide doors and windows that look out into a garden, where I see the disk of the sun rising. I am overcome with a profound sense of lightness and relief.

After the dream was enacted, the protagonist related that she felt like a kind of Egyptian priestess expert in the art of embalming dead bodies. She conveyed the feeling of deep disgust she experienced while she was performing the operation. She had a deep sense of relief when she managed to complete the operation as if she had done a deed that 'had to be done'. She felt that the ritual had the function of 'purification' both for herself and for the body of the dead person, which had to be freed of its 'earthly humours'. When she played the role of the cadaver, she had the feeling that she was something that did not belong to the world of the living any more. (Although the corpse in the dream was hanging by its feet, the protagonist, of course, stood upright while she was playing her role.) Her position in the centre of the room made her feel as if she was the 'central column', a point of reference for the group. She felt she was the transforming centre of the energies that were at work in that context. Another group member associated the dream image with the Hanged Man – the Tarot card that indicates passivity, receptivity and the unalloyed witnessing of ongoing transformations. The cadaver-column at the centre of the room recalls the *djed* column, an object worshipped by the Egyptians as Osiris's body. In its hieroglyphic this column represents the symbol of duration – the cedar of Lebanon that contains the recomposed body of Osiris (Neumann 1993: 231).

In the reflections on the dream and its enactment, regeneration was seemingly connected with people's chances to smear themselves in the cadaver's slimy fluids and in their own dead parts, to face the disgust and horror implicit in it, and to work on putting the body parts together. However, the protagonist concluded that the dream and entire enacted scene was like a kind of 'purification' from material things and 'earthly humours'. Furthermore, she felt that there was both a strong contrast and a complementary relationship between the disgusting aspects of the dissolution of the body and the 'purification of the soul' that she reached in the dream's upstairs room.

In this concluding dream another dismembered cadaver must be put together again in order for people to gain access to their spiritual path.

> I find myself in the amphitheatre classroom for Human Anatomy at the medical school. We are working on putting a cadaver together. There are some colleagues with me, some of whom I recognize as group members. What we are doing is sewing the insides back together to make the supporting structure of a rag doll. Some of us have our hands painted black, others white. When the job is finished, the doll comes alive and I feel that there is something important waiting for me in the street. Looking out the window, I see a procession of rabbis, and I feel like I should join them.

The protagonist was first invited to play the role of himself in the dramatic enactment. At this, he recalled that his hands were painted white in the dream. After this, he was made to exchange roles with a colleague with 'black hands'. He associated white with a 'being in good faith' and black with an 'accepting of compromises' and with 'shadow aspects'. After he enacted the dream, he recognized the complementary nature of the two characters – black-handed and white-handed. He felt that they were linked to two different ways of acting. Both proved to be necessary for him.

He associated this part of the dream with his way of going through his experiences at work. There, 'being painted white too much' made him run the risk of falling into sterile dogmatism. This was something that was certainly imbued with good faith, but ultimately inadequate in real circumstances. So he had to cooperate with characteristics that were more shadowy but more related to the nuts of bolts of his work – 'getting his hands dirty'. This was the only way that the dismembered pieces could be put together again and that the cadaver could come back to life. He related the cadaver to his feelings of depression and impotence in regard to his experiences in the psychiatric work he had recently begun. In this he felt 'fragmented'. The recomposition allowed him to gather up the deepest and most spiritual aspects (the procession of rabbis) that he felt were connected with his professional research. According to Neumann, the preservation and purification of the corpse represent the central core of Osiris's basic mystery – that is, the germination of the spiritual body from the mummified corpse (Neumann 1993: 233).

Chapter 10

Initiatory sickness and ritual suicide

'More or less pathological sicknesses, dreams, and ecstasies are . . . so many means of reaching the condition of shaman', as Eliade reports (Eliade 1974: 33). These means are significant as 'singular experiences' equivalent to initiation ceremonies. As such, they transform an individual profoundly and radically and sharpen his or her intuitive and empathetic potential. The experiences of mystical ecstasy and initiatory sickness that characterize the vocation of the future shaman go through phases more often found in initiation ceremonies – the phases of suffering, death, and resurrection. Whereas initiation ceremonies most often mark the transformation of an adolescent into an adult, initiatory sickness and shamanic ecstasy sanction the transformation of the 'profane man' into a 'technician of the sacred'. Going through both processes, a person encounters suffering, psychological isolation, loneliness, and the feeling of 'immanent death'. These are experienced as a deep transformation of one's own way of being and as something that cannot be undone. Both processes have to do with the double aspect of an earthly and a spiritual path. In this way, the shaman's initiatory sickness takes on a characteristic as a kind of vocation and is experienced as a choice made on high that in some way prepares the candidate for further revelations.

Traces of what Eliade terms 'initiatory sickness' can be found in the dreams, fantasies, and fears of people who come to individual or group analysis in the prospect of working as therapists or of those whose jobs bring them into contact with their own or others' existential disquiet. Of course, the ways in which these sicknesses appear have been adapted to a more rational and less mystical environment with a much dimmer aura of sacredness. People who come to the group seeking therapy but having no professional interest in it can activate within themselves similar traces of fantasies about being initiated into the adult world. If the situation of the professionals recalls shamanic initiation, that of the non-professionals recalls initiation into puberty. The function of the present-day western psychotherapists can be held to be somewhat analogous to that of the shaman of primal peoples, although deprived of the shaman's sacredness. The request for therapy by non-professionals can activate – wittingly or unwittingly – their desires to become more adult and responsible for their own lives. In both categories of people, the 'initiatory sickness' that is encountered in individual and group work is nothing other than the person's own depression.

In a relatively short time, the group puts its members face to face with themselves, with their shadow, and with their potential depression, which cannot remain masked for long. This phase corresponds to entering the *nigredo* in the process of alchemical transformation, as mentioned previously. In the silence that often hangs over the beginning of the sessions, it can happen that participants can question their identity, the motivation that pushed them towards the group, and their more or less taken for granted 'mental health'. Subsequently, serious doubts can begin to come forth.

In this phase, if a person's conscious motivations are strictly professional, these motivations fall away miserably and often make way for a deep existential emptiness that takes their place. Sometimes it may happen that a person can begin to doubt himself or herself by admitting that he or she had been wanting to work as a therapist for some hitherto unexplained motive. This is often expressed as a desire to flaunt one's own sort of standard 'mental health', at least in front of patients who still can be considered much worse off. A person may end up hoping to map out the borders of his or her own mental health. When participants examine their so-called patients' mental processes, they might imagine that they can understand or overcome situations that are related to a kind of suffering and perhaps to their own desperation too, a desperation they can admit neither to others nor themselves. They may admit it, though, by pretending to be referring to others. A participant can ask the group to bring all this to light and make it conscious and acceptable.

These and issues like them have often arisen in the experiences and reflections that doctors, psychologists, and workers in a variety of jobs in the mental health service have brought into groups. Otherwise, when there is a stronger resistance in group work, contents are projected on to conductors, participants, and the group itself as an abstract entity. The group is then experienced as a carrier of chaos, pathology, and confusion as well as a destroyer of structures. Fantasies about contagion emerge, exemplified in some of the dreams of dismemberment treated before and in the following dream.

> Worms are falling off the ceiling. I get the feeling that there is something terribly slimy on me and on the floor. These are the little pieces of the others and of their suffering that are falling on top of me. I am being touched by them and this gradually brings out a reaction of repulsion in me. At the same time I have the feeling that I am dealing with something that can be blocked off even though I sometimes feel the risk of a total invasion.

This dream was related by a health worker, a career nurse, shortly after she was hired by the mental health service. Playing the part of herself in its enactment, the protagonist felt deeply repulsed when she remembered and re-experienced the degrading feeling of the worms falling from the ceiling. She felt that the worms were slimy when they stuck to her and she connected this with an aggressiveness that was hard for her to avoid. Similarly, she felt that many complicated demands and responsibilities were 'raining down on her' from psychiatric patients, colleagues, and institutions in her professional life. On the other hand, she associated the worms that were dropping down from the ceiling with little pieces of other people's life stories, to the sufferings involved in these, and to the emotions and sentiments she felt when dealing with her patients. Similarly, she included the psychodrama group and its members among these associations. As she worked out the dream and the emotions that it involved, she became more and more aware of her own personal suffering, which was at the root of her choice of profession.

The following is the first of two dreams that present vivid illustrations of how becoming a therapist may be linked to an initiation wound.

> I find myself at a tram stop with L. I am going to a psychiatrists' convention. At the entrance there is a sort of electronic machine that checks the identity cards of everybody who wants to go in. I don't have any identity card. I know that the entrance is connected with a sort of 'price to pay'. The machine projects a ray that inflicts a deep wound on all those who don't have their papers in order. This happens to me. This wound will later be treated by a doctor at the convention site itself.

The dreamer was a young female psychologist. L., the man with her at the tram stop, was at that time a gravely ill psychotic patient in a community centre whom she was treating. She had been afraid that she could not 'heal' him 'enough'. When she played the role of this patient (L.), she felt that she had a blind faith in her companion (the dream image of herself) and that she had to put her state of health totally into her therapist's hands. When she played the role of herself, she felt that she could go into the convention only though receiving a kind of 'vaccination' or 'initiation wound' that allowed her to develop her potential for empathy and legitimated her position as therapist. In any case, her wound was attended to at the same place as it was inflicted. The dreamer associated the psychiatric convention with the chance to become a 'technician of healing'. A mythical situation is analogous. Aesculapius, the founder of the medical arts, is said to have been taught medicine by the centaur Chiron, who carried a wound that never healed.

We come across the same theme again with different nuances in this second dream:

> I find myself trudging along in desert terrain towards a group of young people. They look like they are suffering a lot and are full of wounds they do not notice. I feel a strong earthquake tremor and a big crevice opens up in the ground between me and them. I notice that I am now deeply wounded too. The same crevices in the earth are on my body, shaped like wide-open wounds with jagged edges. I am aware that I have to find a road where I can go forward and get past the crevice despite my pain and fatigue. My chances for healing are connected with my chances of reaching 'the other bank'.

The dreamer was a mental health worker at a community for drug addicts, most of whom were HIV positive. He associated the youths on the other bank with his patients. In the dramatic enactment, the protagonist felt that the central issue of the dream was the presence of open wounds, which he recognized as spread equally over his own body, over the drug addicts' bodies, and over the ground in the form of crevices. He associated these wounds with the problem of self-destructiveness and with his difficulty in 'bring the edges of the wounds together' in order to re-link the severed features in his own life. He attributed these wounds to lacerating conflicts that he was rediscovering both in his personal history and career path. Furthermore, he realized that the intense suffering that these conflicts provoked was the source of his ability to enter a deep empathetic relationship with the youths of the centre and so to try to take therapeutic action.

When he played the part of one of the youths, he at first acknowledged that he was deeply distrustful of the participant playing the role of himself as mental health worker. Only the sight of the wounds – which were a kind of identifying mark – overcame his resistance and enabled the youth to get close to the health worker. It also came out into the open during the enactment that the protagonist felt the burning pain of the wounds only when he played the role of himself. When he played the role of one of the 'youths from the other bank', he saw the wounds but did not feel their pain. He associated this phenomenon with the fact that the youths he cared for in the community and who he felt were represented in his dream used heroin as an antidote for their suffering. Heroin took away the pain but did not heal the wounds. The fact that he felt the pain of the conflict upon himself allowed him to be accepted by the youths as a health worker.

He himself was someone who could make the youths aware of a suffering that could make some sense if it was shared. This is what could 'bring the edges of the wound together' and bridge the gap over the crevices in the earth, which he associated with a kind of 'Dantean inferno', gaping with the danger of plummeting down. He recognized this 'inferno' as some of his own destructiveness, which the youths at the centre had chided him for. Therefore the issue he had to work on became clear: he had to become able to stand the suffering inherent in empathetic contact without being overwhelmed by it. In other words, he had to keep a distance as a therapist that would make it possible both for him and the youths to reflect on and work out their problems.

The crevices in this dream that its protagonist associates with the underworld recall Hillman's treatment of the same image. Interestingly enough, Hillman links crevices and the underworld to the sphere of the unconscious:

> Mythology recognized these lacunae in the continuity of ground underfoot, these caves and holes, as entrances to the underworld. Furthermore, like the classical underworld, the unconscious receives mainly a negative description . . . because by definition it is invisible and not directly knowable.
>
> (Hillman 1979: 18)

There are other situations when a sickness could be legitimized by the conscious ego and even become a feature in an image of the persona, hence a kind of social representation or calling card. In this case, the 'sickness' is bound to an external model and therefore tends to lose its own *mana*. While authentic shamanic sickness itself enriches one's sensitivity and potential to see and 'open oneself up to the world', this 'legitimized' sickness becomes a way of shutting oneself off in a protective shell.

The protagonist of the dream we are about to relate exhibited this very feature in her 'sickness'. This was taking place not only in her past but also at the time of her therapy, at least partially. She was a young woman who had been diagnosed as having 'mental anorexia' at the time of her first hospitalization. This syndrome appeared after she suffered a serious trauma in her family just as she was reaching adolescence. At that time, she reacted by rejecting food and enclosing herself inside the 'protective shell' of her sickness. She rotated and is still rotating her entire existence and that of her family members around this protective shell. She was a very sharply and vividly intelligent woman gifted with an acute sense of humour. Despite this, she was never able to place herself into the world of work or construct an autonomous existence for herself. (She was then 35 years old.)

Aside from the way she looked physically – and by then the pathology of her condition was more than apparent – her own self-'diagnosis' was the first thing she showed off like a calling card. 'I am a mental anorexic', she seemed to say to anyone new who would come by. This was the way she introduced herself to the group, where she was quickly accepted, inspiring both interest and sympathy. She even shared several very meaningful episodes from her life with the group, but these were always filtered through her own being 'an anorexic'.

Some time after she entered the group, she showed her first, more marked potential for being approached. In a dream she let a therapist feel her pulse so that she could be treated, but she kept the rest of her body hidden behind the curtain screening off her bed. She associated this scene with the Chinese custom that the emperor's concubines were not supposed to expose themselves to doctors for medical treatment. Instead, they only held out their wrists from behind thick curtains. After the scene was enacted, she said that this was the only way that she felt she could ask for therapeutic intervention – resting hidden 'behind the curtains' she associated with her anorexia.

A short time later, she had the following dream (treated in the section on time):

> I see W. [the woman leader] standing up wrapped like an Egyptian mummy. She is giving oracular answers while falling into a kind of trance. I know that she is living through my anorexia and that she is talking to me about it.

What is happening here is that the sickness has been transferred magically into the therapist just as shamans take on their patients' sickness. Hence the sickness becomes something that the patient transfers into the group leader so that she or he can bring about a transformation connected with healing or with an easing of the symptoms. Thus once the 'sickness as protective shell' or defence is transferred into the therapist, it can change into an initiatory sickness that enables people to open themselves up to the world and thus enhance their sensitivity and heighten their potential for seeing. (In the dream, the therapist gives the patient's anorexia a voice.)

When the dreamer was invited to play the role of the therapist in the dream, she noticed that the sickness inside her had changed. It had been given back to her as her own. She then associated the Egyptian mummy with the 'mummification of her body' – or with the stiffening and shrinking of her bodily senses, sentiments, and emotions. Her emotions had broken out violently and were immediately repressed as her anorexia came on. This followed that very traumatic event that she had witnessed many years before. It was later possible for her to face these emotions and work them out in the group.

Suicides sometimes occur in dreams. Symbolically, they express the renewal and profound regeneration that go along with initiatory sickness. Suicide offers a person a sort of active role regeneration even though it may seem self-destructive. Symbolically it may have something to do with a willing sacrifice of an ego that is static and stiffened. Suicide may symbolize the sacrifice of an old manner of living that has to be abandoned so that a person can progress along his or her individuative path. The image of a symbolic suicide in a dream could thus sanction an entrance into a new existential dimension. In this vein we will re-examine the following dream (seen before in relation to time and to transvestitism) as well as another piece of it that was dreamt later the same night.

> I notice that the little girl is entirely covered with masks, which prevent me even from seeing her face. When she brushes by, passing close to me, the masks fall down suddenly and I notice that they had been covering a void. I feel the presence of the old man, his back turned from me. I feel a very cold feeling. . . .

> I find death by suicide. Maybe I throw myself into a lake and later I find that I am living in a hut at the edge of the forest. I am living frugally but am more closely in tune with nature.

After this latter part of the dream was enacted, the protagonist related that she felt as if she was being 'stripped' of an old identity. All in all, her suicide was not something that was so dramatic but seemed like something that was ritualistic and necessary for her new birth. This new birth proved to be possible and perhaps inevitable after she acknowledged the emptiness at the other side of the masks. She associated this emptiness with the uncovering of something essential that made her aware of a transformation in values. Her new existence was born out of her sacrificing her old one, which she had acknowledged as inauthentic and linked with the masks. This new existence was a 'return to the origins', a seeking for a deeper wellspring of her own essence.

This same theme is found in many fables where a noble-born heroine or hero sacrifices wealth and luxury to seek a new and more authentic sense of existence under more humble appearances, such as *The Goose Girl*, *Sleeping Beauty*, and *Donkey Hide*. This sacrifice can be considered the 'suicide' of the status of outer wealth tied in with the persona, a suicide committed to acquire more deeply meaningful inner values. This theme brings the last chapter of Hermann Hesse's *Steppenwolf* to mind, where the protagonist is asked by figures from his unconscious to commit a 'fake suicide' (Hesse 1963: 242). It is through this 'suicide' that he finally becomes able to understand the world of the 'immortals' and to smile at existence itself.

Chapter 11

The voyage to the underworld

The theme of descent to the underworld or, at least, of encounters with images that belong to the world beyond this one is closely connected with that of the ascent to heaven. This theme is frequently found in initiation processes, shamanic rituals, and myths. The Altaic shaman's voyage to the underworld offers a good example, as Eliade relates:

> The 'black' shaman begins his journey from his own yurt. [Leaving this tent, he then wanders a great deal.] . . . Finally, he reaches the Mountain of Iron, *Temir taixa*, whose peaks touch the sky. It is a dangerous climb; the shaman mimes a difficult ascent, and breathes deeply . . . Once he is across the mountain, another ride takes the shaman to a hole that is the entrance to the other world, *yer mesi*, the 'jaws of the earth', or *yer tunigi*, the 'smoke hole of the earth'.
>
> (Eliade 1974: 201–02)

As Eliade describes, shamanism was important culturally because some of the great themes of the epic emerge in it – especially the voyage to the underworld. These were to be taken up again in various literary traditions (Eliade 1974: 213). Experiences involving the same themes on the symbolic level turn up frequently in fairy tales and dreams.

The voyage to the underworld has been imagined in various ways. First, it can be seen as a journey down into a subterranean world, which is made up of caves pointing towards a hypothetical centre of the earth and following the line of the *axis mundi*. Second, it can be seen as a voyage on the water towards the open sea or towards far-away islands of the dead. Such a voyage can progress down underground rivers or through spaces in the air. Third, it can be seen as movements made not by the protagonist himself or herself, but by the souls of the dead who appear to him or her in dreams and visions. Fourth (and not last), it can be seen as an encounter with an enigmatic figure who turns out to be a personified image of death (a theme running through many of the dreams discussed).

THE DESCENT INTO THE BOWELS OF THE EARTH

As Eliade describes, a person descends into the underworld in flesh and blood, faces monsters and hellish demons, and goes through an initiatory test whose goal is often the conquest of bodily immortality. Many myths and fairy tales describe the entrance into the bowels of the earth and the underworld as a process of being eaten by a monstrous beast whose wide open jaws are like the entrance to a cave or the gates of hell. Groping about inside the bowels of the beast corresponds to wandering about in the labyrinthine world of the shadows. The protagonist can be born again to a new life only if he or she finds the way out. This is exemplified in some of the variant episodes of the *Kalevala*. In it the wise man Vainamoinen goes on a voyage to the land of the dead where he is swallowed by the daughter of Tuoni, the lord of the world beyond. When he reaches the giant woman's stomach, he builds a boat, begins to row briskly, and so forces her to vomit him up into the sea (Eliade 1965: 62ff.).

The following dream expresses clearly how the pathway through the underworld can be experienced as a labyrinth. It was narrated by a new participant shortly after joining the group.

I find myself holding a very weak torch inside a cave. A little bit farther on, I reach a kind of circular room where many mineshafts begin. They seem to be labyrinthine paths that criss-cross and split into two continuously. I meet figures who seem like shadows and are involved in looking for solitary routes for themselves. The features of their faces keep on changing just as soon as I feel that I am about to recognize them.

The dreamer associated the people she met with some of the group members and with aspects of herself that they had commented to her about. When she played the role of herself in the enactment, she first felt disoriented, shortly afterwards she overcame this feeling, and finally replaced it with an intense fascination for the 'labyrinthine world'. The dreamer related that she had had the feeling that the torchlight allowed her to perceive eventual dangers but that at the same time it was weak enough to let her eyes get used to the darkness. This allowed her to discover a very unusual way of seeing that she associated with the situation she was experiencing with the group. There she had given up on 'seeing herself and the others' in bright light. In other words, she stopped trying to understand everything and everybody in the light of rational consciousness. She had become able to 'get used to the weaker light'. Now she could gather in intuitions and feelings that were hardly noticeable before and begin to make out the darker and lighter sides of her world of relationships.

When the dreamer played the role of some of the people she had met and identified as parts of herself, she related that the penumbra allowed their profiles and expressions to keep on changing, but that she had nevertheless become capable of finding a stable identity in the group. She also related that she had gained the positive option of facing changes by getting herself out of the static and stereo-typical roles that she felt she had been imprisoned in. In any case, she associated all this with her fatiguing effort to find her own way in her life in a situation marked by a penumbra where she could neither recognize nor be certain of anything.

The numerous labyrinthine designs traced out on the sand at Malekula are of interest in relation to the dream above and to the theme of initiation in the under-world, as Eliade explains, drawing from the research of Deacon and Layard:

> [the designs] . . . have the purpose of teaching the road to the abode of the dead. In other words, the labyrinth consists in a postmortem initiatory test. It is one of the obstacles that the dead person – or the hero, in other cases – must face in his voyage to the world beyond. Here it should be emphasized that the labyrinth presents itself as a dangerous passage towards the bowels of mother earth, where the soul of the dead person runs the risk of being eaten by a female monster. . . . The other world widens its borders more and more. It no longer means only the land of the dead. It means every enchanted and miraculous sign and, by extension, both the divine and the transcendent world. The 'toothed vagina' is liable to represent not only the passage towards the interior of 'mother earth', but also the gate of heaven.
>
> (Eliade 1965: 62, 66; Deacon 1934)

The following dream illustrates a descent into the bowels of the earth (and will be taken up later in relation to the elements of earth and fire).

> I feel strongly attracted by a cave whose mouth I see. I venture to go into its depths and I make out a stretch of sand on the inside that I had not noticed before. It is glowing weakly. Suddenly I notice that my mother is next to me. She shows me some sparks of fire on the sand. She explains that if you blow on the sparks, they change into fires and materialize into images of warriors.

The dreamer's mother had been dead for several years at the time of the dream. She was a woman who was intensely fascinating to her daughter. She said that her mother seemed to be omnipotent, but had some deeply troubling traits. Her mother had given birth 12 times and had terminated an indefinite number of other preg-nancies with abortions. The dreamer was the youngest child and was bound to her mother by very intense affection, but she felt deeply inferior to her. Her mother's extraordinary fertility held the daughter in great awe of her and she always felt crushed by her in some way. Similarly, her mother's ability to give and reabsorb life within herself disquieted her deeply. She felt so crushed and limited by an overpowering image of femininity that she really felt as if she had been castrated. As she was leading her life, the dreamer had constantly been struggling to mark out a sphere of autonomy for herself, which she felt was always being threatened. Her struggle forced her to leave home at too early an age and sacrifice some important aspects of her femininity.

At the time of the dream, the protagonist was going through a period of depression and was working out her relationship with her mother in individual and group analysis. This dream marked an important turning point in her progress, starting from the moment when it was possible for her to enter the cave with her mother without being sucked into her or devoured. She finally became able to feel enlivened by the presence of a mother who was no longer threatening. She could now take energy and courage from her – appearing in the form of the souls of the materialized warriors. This is what she needed to face her professional life and her inner searching in a more decisive way – a stance that she associated with the sparks under the sand. As Eliade relates, shamans usually travel to the underworld in order to find the sick person's lost or escaped soul, lead it back to the kingdom of the living, and work a magical cure. Sometimes, instead, they may do the opposite, like the Altaic area shamans, who 'escort the soul of the deceased to Erlik's realm', the realm of the Altaic underworld god (Eliade 1974: 203). In the dream above we can consider the lost soul as the soul of the woman dreamer, which can be seen as the life energy that is rediscovered in the warriors that materialize from the sparks.

UNDERGROUND WATER AND THE OPEN SEA

I find myself in a cave that ends in a corridor leading to three rooms. In one of these, there is a raised area that has a mummy of a woman on it, maybe my mother. I try to give her some orders: 'Get up', 'Walk', 'Speak'. She follows the orders mechanically. She sits and starts to look like an oracle. I ask her about myself and my son, but she does not answer me. I notice that an underground river is gushing in the room. Then other female figures reach this place and they are all essentially the same figure, but they have various shapes and features.

The protagonist was invited to play the role of herself and that of the mummy in the dramatic enactment. As the mummy, she recognized her own feminine side and affections, which she had mummified by trying to hold them under control. This made her see the problems she had in trying to relate to the world in a 'feminine' way – that is, being receptive and welcoming. This was something that came out in her personal life, where her mummified emotions prevented her from reacting in a meaningful way. However, when she then played the role of the mummy, she also felt that she could 'hear' what was happening inside the world of the caves 'and above it'. Above all, she felt that she could 'tune in on' the moods of the people that came close to her. She associated her oracular aspects with a kind of 'secret consciousness' that she attributed to the dead because they were detached from the everyday world.

Many religions and myths describe the world beyond as a place of knowledge and wisdom. In fact, the lords of the underworld are often omniscient and the dead seem to know the future. In dreams they often have this function. In some myths and sagas, the hero goes into the underworld to get wisdom or to obtain secret knowledge. In her reading of the fairy tale, 'The Three Feathers', the Jungian scholar Marie-Louise von Franz observes that its hero does not waste his energy on surface matters in an effort to look for banal solutions, as his brothers do. Instead, he 'went down into the earth' (Franz 1996: 46ff.; Grimm 1969: tale 63). He goes down through a trap door and descends a ladder that takes him underground to the frog-queen. He takes her treasures from this underground kingdom and these allow him to inherit the kingdom. As Hillman observes, the underworld is a community with countless members (Hillman 1979: 41). The infinite varieties of the figures present reflect the infinity of the soul. Dreams give this sense of multiplicity back to the consciousness and this is perhaps what was happening in the dream narrated above.

As emerged in the protagonist's associations, she was asking the group to help her rediscover the element of wetness running somewhere through the underworld – the underground water that could make a transformation possible. At the same time, it seemed that she looked to the springs of renewal that gushed out of the depths as a way of 'finding the answers' to the questions that were being raised as she was moving about the world.

In the preceding sections we have seen how coming into the group often corresponds symbolically to being torn up and rent to pieces by the group itself. However, coming into a group can also correspond to being taken into the belly of the whale and warming oneself with the heat of the blood that is beating – that is, a *regressio ad uterum*, a step-by-step return to a symbiotic, uroboric state. Here there is the risk of getting lost in the multifarious labyrinths that are revealed as one person encounters another. However, there is also the chance for a person to be enriched in an infinite number of new routes and existential possibilities. He or she can encounter the underworld river – the water of life that can dissolve and transform his or her own mummified aspects and reveal newer and newer oppor-tunities in them. He can nourish himself from the heart of the animal (the 'whale' he may be inside), as we have seen in the section on the sacred meal. As in every analytical process, in the group this feeling corresponds to a person's attraction towards dependence, as well as his fear of it. It is a chance for transformation, but also for claustrophobia. It is the feeling of being closed inside an alchemist's vessel of transformation. These and experiences like them are often expressed by group members in their dreams and their reflections in the group.

Group members have expressed the barriers that they had to pass through in order to reach the 'open sea' in terms of the 'Columns of Hercules', 'Symplegades', and 'Caudine Forks'. (The first two are ancient terms for the Straits of Gibraltar. The third is part of a proverbial Italian expression that means 'running the gauntlet', named for a narrow mountain pass in southern Italy, site of a Roman army's defeat.) The following dream is an example:

> I am sailing on an ancient Greek vessel with sails spread out towards the open sea through the Columns of Hercules or the Symplegades. The crew is mute. The 'utensils of the giants' who belong to a preceding epoch of the titans are

floating on the water as well as a broken column. There is also a gigantic 'royal duck' who first seems dead but is really only asleep. What strikes me is the intense light blue of the sky, the sea, and the breast of the royal duck, each of which is a different shade of blue.

In the associations, the 'utensils of the giants' represented the elements of rough and archaic everyday life that have been abandoned. These have to be left behind and passed by in order to reach the 'Columns of Hercules' and face the open sea. In the enactment the sleeping or falsely dead royal duck was identified as an element that belonged to the air and the water, a bird that is able to fly towards transcendence. The duck probably gets its life back and wins the right to 'fly to the heights' as it passes the place where the giants' utensils have been caught up or smashed.

The passage through the straits is described by Eliade as a kind of ability to fly into another state.

> The Symplegades show us the paradoxical nature of the passage into the beyond, or, more precisely, of transfer from this world into a world that is transcendent. For although originally the other world was the world after death, it finally comes to mean any transcendent state.
>
> (Eliade 1965: 65)

When the group exposes the bare surface of its own contradictions, when it allows burning conflicts to emerge, and when it brings opposing and contradictory desires, thoughts, and feelings to light, it then exhibits its vain titanic struggles. Through its own suffering, the group holds up to its conscious mind the enigmas and conflicts that can never be resolved on a human and rational level. Everything changes and moves constantly. If a person does not recognize these changes and does not admit that he or she cannot resolve these enigmas on a human and rational level, he or she will inevitably be crushed by them and forced to backtrack and limit his or her horizons. A person can pass through these 'straits' – through the 'Columns of Hercules' with their crashing massive rocks – only if he or she recognizes them as a passage towards the world of the transcendent. This seemed to be the message of the dream.

If this recognition does not happen, what emerges in the psychodrama group is what can become the uncrossable border of 'stopping at the concrete level', of 'interpreting literally' without passing on towards an imaginative symbolic level. In this way, what come out of the conflicts and contents are merely the personal and relational features of these conflicts. In other words, the royal duck can keep on sleeping and forget its chance to fly, thereby running the risk of being crushed. A person runs the risk of feeling uniquely rent asunder by the 'Symplegades' – the 'straits' of the conflicts –without going on to pass through into the more-than-personal archetypal contents that underlie them. Eliade writes about how the Symplegades make a kind of initiatory selection. They separate those who cannot detach themselves from immediate reality from those who discover freedom of the spirit, the chance to free themselves from material laws through thought. He states:

> The Symplegades become in some sort 'guardians of the threshold', homolo-
> gizable with the monsters and griffins that guard a treasure hidden at the
> bottom of the sea, or a miraculous fountain from which flows the Water of
> Youth.
>
> (Eliade 1965: 66)

The imagination, fantasy and intuition are activated when they are catalysed in the group while dreams are evoked and scenes are enacted. This gives a group member the chance to develop his or her receptiveness and openness towards infinite opportunities. All this makes it possible for him or her to 'fly' – i.e. to perform a creative act in order to overcome the barriers and tensions between opposites.

DEPTH, ABYSS, VOID

According to Hillman, Tartaros has been imagined as the extreme depth of Hades from the time of Hesiod on. It was compared to the firmament and personified as a son of the sky and the earth – that is, a kingdom of dust, a mix of the material and the immaterial. Dreams, which belong to the world of Hades, 'must refer to a psychic or pneumatic world of ghosts, spirits, ancestors, souls, daimones' (Hillman 1979: 38–39). The dream appears to be a fluid – dusty, fiery, muddy or airy – space. There is nothing solid to hang on in its sphere. Only intuition can brush by something impalpable that slips between a person's fingers or burns up as soon as he or she touches it.

In psychodrama groups, the ghosts, spirits, ancestors and daimones that are already there in the dream world gain strength and number. They contact and summon each other while they are being encouraged by participants who are enacting their projections and expectations. When the participants explore the frontiers of the soul and the dream world, they find themselves – sometimes surprisingly – in contact with a void without limits. In this way, the world of the soul opens its abysses, its depths, and unexpected chasms. This process thus appears to be an inexhaustible journey beyond any reality that the senses can conceive, a journey that reflects Heraclitus's search for a soul without limits that delves deeper and deeper in its search for an 'invisible and hidden harmony' (Heraclitus 1969: fragment 51).

This group member's dream shows the 'pneumatic' or airy aspect of the underworld.

> I go down a wooden ladder and arrive at the centre of the earth. Here the
> air has become rarefied and it is no longer possible to make out the line of
> the horizon. I mount a winged animal that reminds me of Geryon in Dante's
> *Inferno*. As I fly, I realize that the animal has the face of the group leader.

Here the dreamer expects the therapist to be able to guide her through the depths. She is attributed with some characteristics of the shaman-bird, a figure often encountered in North American mythology (Eliade 1974: 164). At the same time she is also a creature of the underworld that participates in it. This is analogous to a dream that will soon be examined in which the woman group leader represents the semblance of death.

According to a Yakut legend from Siberia, there is a giant spruce in the north that has nests on its branches (Eliade 1974: 37). A magic bird with the head of an eagle and iron feathers lays eggs and sits on them. The shamans originate from these eggs. The motif of the giant bird that hatches shamans on the branches of the tree of the world is of great importance in the various north Asian mythologies. Sometimes even unborn babies are birds roosting on trees where shamans look for them. The theme of the tree and the bird is often present in dreams about the shamanic vocation. The motif of the shaman as a bird is closely connected with the image of being carried into the kingdom of the dead.

> . . . in the imagination of late antiquity Tartaros was a region of dense cold air without light. Hence, Hades was often spoken of as having wings, just as in the Gilgamesh Epic, Enkidu dreams of his death as a transformation into a bird, his arms covered with feathers. The dead are clad like birds, their element evidently air.
>
> (Hillman 1979: 38)

Thus this theme features the bird as emblem of apparent death and possible resurrection through the soul and spirit. The royal duck from the dream of passing through the Columns of Hercules is one example. The following dream offers another: 'As I go down, I notice that feathers are growing on my arms and that maybe my arms themselves are changing into wings. . . . Other birds are flying around me.'

The image of the soul transformed into a bird is present in various mythologies. Thus the soul becomes something that can fly and, free of the body, can rise towards the heavens. A bird in flight, symbol of the soul that is directed towards heaven, is represented on the funeral pillars in some villages in Transylvania (Cook 1974: 127, plate 95). Several authors narrate that the body of the dead pharaoh is transported on the wings of the sacred ibis, Thoth. The flight on a bird's back is cited in the *Egyptian Book of the Dead* itself (Propp 1985: 331ff.). This theme is also found in Tahiti, in Oceania, in northwestern American mythology, in Babylonia, and in classical antiquity. The image of the soul-bird may have originated in the representation picturing the soul as rising with the smoke while its body was being cremated. In Artemidorus's treatise on dreams, every bird that appears in the dream world is interpreted as a man. Further, every flight is interpreted as the aspiration of the soul to cast off its earthly mantle by flying in the Elysian fields in the form of a bird–animal, a theme to be covered again in the section on the element of air. Finally, birds often appear in fairy tales in relation to the representation of the world of the spirit, a far-away world that the hero can reach. In fact, the bird is linked to the earth because it dwells on trees, but it has the chance to free itself in the air. This allows it to reach infinite spaces. The bird as transporter to the world beyond is found most often among peoples living on coastlines.

To return to the previously related dream, the protagonist had just entered the group and brought in her issues around this. She had trouble trying to enter the world of symbols, tuning in on them, and distancing herself from the more concrete aspects of reality that she felt imprisoned in. She then associated the other birds in flight, whose metamorphoses seemed to have been completed, with the other group members whom she perceived as 'able to fly'.

DEATH AS A CHARACTER AND A SYMBOL

Russian fairy tales often tell of a hut mounted on a hen's foot at the edge of a forest that can twist and rotate around its central axis. The hut is situated along a closed, uncrossable border and its entrance opens into the world of the dead, which the fairy tale hero can only get out of by flying. The hut is often the dwelling of super-natural beings – most often of a witch, Baba Yaga, and of figures associated with her. Here is an example related by Propp:

> At one point, the geese-shamans had to fly in the sky through an opening. An old woman who was watching the geese that were flying by sat next to this opening . . . No living man can fly in this area. The Lord of the Universe does not allow it.
>
> (Propp 1985: 95ff.)

The old woman stays to watch over the entrance to the kingdom of the dead. She represents death itself. In this type of fairy tale, the hero is not a dead person, but a living man or shaman who wants to break into the kingdom of the dead. As is known, the fairy tale as initiation is connected to the theme of the journey to the world beyond – the world below or the world above. The beginnings of the tales often present encounters with characters that evoke representations of death. The fence around the witch's hut is made of human bones and its roof is studded with skulls with their eyes intact. Propp relates:

> The magic woman in the hut that is too small recalls a dead body in a tight coffin or in a little casket where someone is buried. She often has bony legs that mark her skeletal aspect and her membership in the kingdom of death.
>
> (Propp 1985: 112ff.)

At other times the magic woman is presented as a figure who seduces, charms, and entraps the hero, attracting him towards the kingdom of the dead. This is exem-plified by the elf queen of Anglo-Saxon legends as well as by sirens and 'Melusinas' (dark sea witches) who hide their fish or serpent tails that betray their underground origins. The elf queen also makes her appearances in the heart of the forest. The sirens and the 'rusalkas' (mermaids) of the Russian fairy tales are found at the borders of the earth and the water, while the Melusinas reign over the borders between earthly depths and the surface world.

Female figures who share characteristics with the elves, sirens and rusalkas often turn up in dreams.

> I am walking with R. along some rocks besides a stormy sea. In the distance I see a very thin woman dressed in black on the sea's edge. When I approach her, I see that she is burning sea urchin shells to keep herself warm.

The protagonist chose the group leader to play the role of the woman in black. She was then invited to exchange roles with her. She associated the woman in black with death. When she herself played that role, she felt she was a sort of divinity or mythical character who intended to perform a ritual that aimed to give a significant message about sacrifice and transformation. She said that R., the dream companion at her side, reminded her of a problem with self-destructiveness that she was confronting at that time. The sea urchins were associated with elements from the depths of the sea that could wound and get under the skin, and were hard to extract. The dreamer associated the fire with the chance to burn household rubbish, as is done in the country, but here the fire became a sacrificial fire.

Hillman reminds us that household rubbish was sacred to Hekate, the three-headed underworld goddess that sanctifies what is discarded in the everyday world. According to the ritual, the rubbish was deposited at a crossroads every night. Even dreams can be seen in this light in as much as they can be considered the leftovers of the day – or as Freud defined them, the 'scraps' of daily life (Hillman 1979: 40–41ff.) Hekate is the goddess who, like a dream, allows us to see and listen in many ways at the same time. The crossroads where she is offered sacrifices can lead in three directions besides the direction a person is coming from, perhaps symbolized in Hekate's three heads turned in different directions. Actually, the problem that the dreamer brought forward in relation to her self-destructiveness could only be faced through the eyes of Hekate in order to get her past a dead end that she could not have gone beyond otherwise.

The following dream deals more explicitly with death characterized as transformation and the way the death symbol is projected on to the group leader, who becomes an emblem of the initiatory-analytic process:

> I find myself stopped at a railroad crossing in front of double crosses of St Andrew. A little bit later, I find myself in the psychodrama group and I realize that W., the group leader, has the features of death.

The dreamer associated the St Andrew's cross (that is found on road signs at unguarded railway crossings) with a warning and with the fear of being run over. Correspondingly he said he sometimes felt run over by the psychodrama group, which was a totally new and unnerving experience for him in respect to his earlier way of life. The symbol represented something positive about a synthesis between rural life (the St Andrew's cross sign that is often found in the country) and city life (the train that links different cities). The rural aspect could be linked to his rediscovery of his roots and of his more 'visceral' features in the group through his psychodramatic work. The city aspect could be linked to his more 'civilized' and rationalizing part, the part more 'of his head'.

Although the group leader was deeply disquieting as death, she held out the image of the rhythmic beating of time and of deep transformation. This image could be connected to the chance the protagonist was being given to change and renew himself. As in the previously mentioned dream of Geryon, the image of the therapist as a figure with shamanic characteristics has made another appearance. In fact, one of the most important initiatory tests that is common among both Siberian and Eskimo shamans consists in the contemplation of their own skeletons. The same practice is found in some Buddhist and tantric meditations that Eliade has written extensively about. Here the reduction to the state of a skeleton has a prevailingly ascetic and metaphysical value. It is the equivalent of anticipating the workings of time on the body and of using one's thoughts to break life down to what it really is: 'an ephemeral illusion in perpetual transformation' (Eliade 1974: 63).

Chapter 12

The passage through the elements

An essential moment in every esoteric path is the passage of the initiate through the elements. The philosopher Gaston Bachelard maintains that the four physical elements are analogous to four different types and temperaments. He underlines their differences and antagonisms:

> . . . it seems quite clear to us that there is some relation between the doctrine of the four physical elements and the doctrine of the four temperaments . . . Indeed, the tetravalence of reverie is as clear and productive as the chemical tetravalence of carbon. Reverie has four domains, four points from which it soars into infinite space . . . 'Tell me what your favorite phantom is. Is it the gnome, the salamander, the sylph or the undine?' Now – and I wonder if this has been noticed – all these chimerical beings are formed from and sustained by a unique substance: the gnome, terrestrial and condensed, lives in the fissure of the rock, guardian of the mineral and the gold, and stuffs himself with the most compact substances; the salamander, composed all of fire, is consumed in its own flame; the water nymph or undine glides noiselessly across the pond and feeds on her own reflection; the sylph for whom the least substance is a burden, who is frightened away by the tiniest drop of alcohol, who would even perhaps be angry with a smoker who might 'contaminate her element' (Hoffmann), rises effortlessly into the blue sky, happy in her anorexia.
>
> (Bachelard 1964: 89–90)

EARTH

The earth has often been associated symbolically with wealth and the resources of the land. Money, the medium of exchange of wealth, is the image of material values, and it can also symbolize energy, spiritual and affective value, and interior potential. Entering a psychodrama group or working in analysis often means coming to terms with one's own values and comparing these with other values, comparing them with one another, and measuring their exchange rate against the group's 'hard currency' – i.e. the prevailing values that the group consciously and unconsciously uses as its medium of exchange. Some participants dream that they find themselves penniless or with a soft foreign currency. Some feel that they find they have a valuable currency in a country where it is not honoured. Yet there are others who ask help from the group and from the work of analysis so that they can find the pieces of gold that they had and that are now hidden under the earth or in an unknown place. The protagonist in the following dream is one of these. She had the dream after she participated in a psychodrama session. Its symbolic use of money and the earth is of interest.

> At last I went away from that dingy, bare room and reached the garden. Here the gardener invited me to dig in the tilled soil under a plant. Various bracelets and gold jewels came out linked together. He asked me if I recognized anything that belonged to me, but unfortunately it seemed that none of them had ever belonged to me. For a moment I was tempted to lie and take someone else's things unfairly, but I didn't have the courage to do it.

In the enactment of the dream, the protagonist associated her leaving the room in order to go into the garden with her need to get away from her usual way of being, at least for a time. This way seemed extinguished and lifeless and she wanted to get in touch again with the natural element represented by the earth. She chose the male group leader for the role of the gardener. She was then invited to switch roles and play the role of the gardener. She felt that she was representing an internal figure that she associated with the group leader, whose job it was to accompany each person in the hunt for 'one's own treasure' – i.e. a sort of family legacy that represented something very personal.

However, the hunt was not so simple and it involved bringing other people's treasures to light and learning how to distinguish them from her own. She associated her desire to take other people's gold coins unfairly with a problem of the persona, or with her desire to 'appear' to herself and others as a person who had the values she would have liked to have. She herself had been projecting these values on to the group, so she did not feel that they were her own. After the enactment, she added that during the scene she had the feeling that she would have found what she was looking for in the earth not too far away from where she was.

The earth is entrusted with the ability to produce riches. It can enclose, receive, contain, and transform. The riches may be material – harvest, grains, vegetation, etc. – or the symbolic wealth of energetic values. These are protected, guarded, incubated, or hidden; or they are even dug up and brought into the daylight. Hence the psychodrama group takes on the features of a piece of symbolic earth that reflects the earth of each group member. Here exploration, excavation, and searching is possible because others help dig into the earth. This earth becomes an observation point where the seeds sown in times gone by are found again and where seeds of one's own can be sown and wait to be transformed. This aspect is evident in the following dream.

> I am walking in woods and I see a lot of holes dug in the earth. There is something deeply unnerving in the air. In one of the holes I see the body of an unweaned infant. He is very pale and seems to be dead. A little further up I see another one like him. I feel that I have to get them out of the holes, but I don't do it. I take my camera and fix their images in a photograph.

Here the tilled soil is connected with the individual and group analytical work that the woman dreamer had recently undertaken. The holes were unnerving because they recalled something buried, perhaps prematurely, and brought up images of interment. In the dramatization of the dream the protagonist was invited to play the role of herself and of the newborn infants. In her reflections later, she identified the infants as the double chance to grow creatively that had been buried prematurely along with her 'joy in living'. She herself was surprised and upset when the infants appeared, but she did not feel like observing them more closely or bringing them to light. She perhaps was afraid to find herself in front of two asphyxiated corpses. She limited herself to taking their pictures and the dream ended there.

The memory of this dream turned up again in her analytical work several months later. She had been having trouble choosing between two opportunities and was afraid of missing out on both. The protagonist then associated this problem with a dream that followed, which came to mind because it also involved a camera. The only thing that she remembered was that there was a shining star and that she could not make its image stand still by taking its picture. After this she realized that the infants of the earlier dream were really alive but very deeply asleep. The idea began to take hold of her that the infants could regain their colour and become alive again once they were brought out into the light. However, they needed something active – a direct perceiving and feeling that could reactivate their circulation and make their blood flow again. Skin contact had to substitute the camera.

In her associations, all this seemed to represent the first phase in the process of transformation that she was undergoing in analysis. In the first dream the infants may have been buried prematurely in the earth and could only be seen and photographed. She could note their existence, but the time was not ripe for them to be touched or for anyone even to imagine that she could reach out and touch them. Only in the following phase of maturity could they transform themselves. Only then could people notice that they were not dead but just pale from never having seen the sunlight. They were like shoots that are just as colourless as long as they stay under the soil. At the same time the dreamer recognized that the infants may have been hidden, but they were also guarded, in the receptive and welcoming lap of mother earth.

What the dreamer recognized is somewhat similar to the analogy that the ancient Egyptians drew between the body in the earth and the seed that is to bloom later. Eliade writes of their rituals:

> Through certain rituals the Egyptians created an 'agricultural fate' for the soul of the dead person by transforming it into a seed. The body is made to return to the great womb of Tellus, the source of all forms.

> (Eliade 1989: 213)

The earth may be seen as a place of receptivity, welcome, and burial. However, it is also a place where concrete actions have the chance to be transformed. A group member expressed such an image of the earth in a dream that she narrated shortly after her entry into the group.

> I find myself at the entrance of a cemetery and I observe a common ossuary in front of me, where a mountain of bones are piled up and mixed up together. A little farther ahead there are some bulldozers that are in the middle of some work in progress. They are turning over the soil and, when they dig holes, they bring a lot of bones to light, which seem to belong to different historical epochs. They have to make space for the burial of the more recent dead.

Here a pile recurs as a dream image, something similar to the pile of clothes in a dream discussed earlier in relation to transvestitism. This pile was associated with the psychodrama group as the dream was being dramatized. However, this time bones – not clothes – are heaped together. Whereas clothes just cover the body's surface, bones go deeper. They represent a more archaic and profound past and are more strictly connected with the very essence of the body.

In the dream discussed in relation to transvestitism, the piled-up and exchanged clothes gave the group members ways of bringing into the light their roles in life and some facets of their personas. The psychodrama group gave its members the room to try on the roles along with the clothes that they were putting on in order to present themselves to the world and to themselves. Besides this, they could test out their emotional responses to what they were doing. In the cemetery dream something else is going on. The bones in the ossuary and the bones uncovered by the bulldozers that turned over the soil seem to relate to deeper and more ancient material than the clothes. These bones are linked with archetypes of the collective unconscious. Yet, the group is also the 'earth' surface, where what was hidden and buried since time immemorial is stirred up again. It is the place where 'the ancestors' bones' and the 'skeletons in the closet' come out into the light again.

A person's own roots lie in the 'ancestors' bones'. So does the very essence of human nature. So does the essence of his or her own nature, which is different from, yet similar to, those of the others. Here the bones recall the 'reduction down to the bone' that the shaman undergoes. The saying 'skeletons in the closet' indicates that a person has something in himself that he has gone beyond and that is long dead, something burdensome and useless, something that he may want to hide. There is often something blameworthy that is held hidden and that had better be brought out into the light. The group seemed to see to it that all these things would happen.

The same theme of the earth as a cemetery – a place of the burial and reception of essences that are to be put together and harmonized – is expressed in the following dream. At the beginning the protagonist realizes that she has found herself in a submarine.

I realized that it was river water that I was dealing with and that the submarine was surfacing from under the Seine at Paris, where it left us off. Here I suddenly found myself alone in a gigantic square, where many streets came together like spokes on a wheel. I recognized it as *Place de la Concorde*. I had the impression that the name was important and the structure of the square was rather different than the way I remembered it in reality. I was impressed by the streets' spoke-like layout, which had the look of a mandala. Little by little the landscape transformed itself and at last I found myself in the Monumental Cemetery in Turin, where several boulevards converge. At the centre there is the monument to Tamagno [a Turin musician].

In the dramatization of the dream the protagonist felt an intense emotion when she played the part of the statue of Tamagno. She said later that something everlasting emanated from it because it was sculpted in stone yet alive. She began to fantasize that the monument was situated on top of the ossuary of a common grave (this is not true in reality) and that its function was to harmonize the souls with the orchestra conductor's baton, transforming their discordant sounds into harmony.

When the dream was brought into the reality of the psychodrama group, she revealed that it had aroused her conflicting emotions, states of mind, and fantasies in her current analytical work. These were things that belonged to such long-gone periods of her life that she believed she had buried them a long time ago. Something deeper and more essential emerged that she connected with the nakedness of the bones, something that was individual and collective at the same time. It was now up to her to deal with the problem of putting all of this together.

The image of 'mother earth' who receives and harmonizes bodies and souls is often strictly connected with the image of a feminine figure that encounters the archetype of the Great Mother. Goethe describes such an image as 'the Mothers'.

> Dwelling in eternal obscurity and loneliness, these Mothers are creative beings; they are the creating and sustaining principle from which proceeds everything that has life and form on the surface of the earth. Whatever ceases to breathe returns to them as a spiritual nature, and they preserve it until there arises occasion for its renewed existence.
>
> (Goethe 1951: 342)

Goethe calls this the eternal metamorphosis of the earthly existence of being born, growing, transforming and destroying oneself.

There is a particularly pregnant image in the following dream (treated before in relation to the underworld). Here the earth is featured as the hardness of the rock in which a welcoming cave is dug out, where we find the woman dreamer.

> I feel strongly attracted by a cave whose mouth I see. I venture to go into its depths and I make out a stretch of sand on the inside that I had not noticed before. It is glowing weakly. Suddenly I notice that my mother is next to me.

> She shows me some sparks of fire on the sand. She explains that if you blow
> on the sparks, they change into fires and materialize into images of warriors.

We will return to the nature of the 'sparks' later when treating the element of fire. Here we will concentrate on the archetype and the associations related to the image of the mother. The mother had evoked an intense fascination in the dream's protagonist. She said her mother had some omnipotent qualities, but that these went along with some deeply disquieting features. (Chapter 11 dealt with some aspects of the mother's troubled relationship with the dreamer.) In this context, the theme of mother earth is taken up again in the symbol of the cave and in the presence of a feminine figure that has the characteristics of the Great Mother. The dream also associates the warriors and the Great Mother.

Astarte, the prime Semitic goddess, is the divine protectress of love and of universal fertility as well as of warriors. Nanaia, a goddess worshipped in Mesopotamia and Iran, is a divine warrior. She is called on by soldiers in combat and invoked by kings seeking victory against their enemies. Ishtar was also a goddess of fertility and war from very ancient times in Babylonia (Eliade 1989: 17). Like these goddesses, the group shares in the protective, nourishing, and welcoming qualities of the Great Mother. It evokes 'warrior spirits' to support each member's process of individuation, above all when a person takes on some of the obstacles that may block his or her path of individuation.

In the dramatization, the protagonist was invited to play the role of the sparks on the sand. It was then that she recognized the importance of feeling that she was 'contained and protected' by the environment and the group, so that she could find the energy and the courage necessary to take up her personal battles in her familial, emotional, and professional environments. She related the blowing, which was claimed to transform the sparks, to the intervention of an internal masculine figure who made himself the activator of the process.

This dream contains motifs treated elsewhere. It describes a progression like the herb warrior's in the sacred meal section. It shows the group as the potentially threatening and devouring Great Mother earth described in the ritual dismemberment section. It features the earth as a cave, something also seen in the section on the underworld.

The earth in the group is also its base of support, the concrete element that everyone is brought to measure themselves against. The earth is the position a person assumes in relation to his or her own ground and sky. It is the need and the chance for a person to make his projections touch the ground and be measured against 'the other' in his physical presence, in his bodily and psychic reality and in the immediacy of his connections with the here and now. In its psychic and physical space, the group embodies and traces out an earth *temenos* to refer to at a set time, a home base against which a person can redefine and reorder his whole world, his interior images, and his vision of the world. Although the group evokes the image of the earth as base and as the chance to touch and face reality, it may simultaneously evoke the opposite – loss of contact with the reality of everyday life. The following dream expresses both aspects of a group.

> I find myself with others at the passage out of a temple at the end of a religious function. It is probably a Moslem or Hindu holy place, where you can enter only if you take off your shoes. In the space in front of the exit the shoes and sandals of very many of the faithful have been deposited. I look for mine without finding them.

In the session before the protagonist related this dream, many other dreams were enacted. In this session he linked the religious function to the group. Inner images and the search for innerness took up space in the group, but sometimes seemed to overwhelm everyday reality. He recognized himself from among the faithful because he felt deeply enriched by the path he had taken up, by the images of the soul, and by the dreams that the psychodrama sessions were stimulating. He associated his taking off his shoes in the temple with the chance to contact the earth more directly and intensely with the soles of his bare feet with nothing in between. Yet, the intensity that the feelings evoked in him made him afraid to re-enter the 'everyday world' without shoes. When he lost or was robbed of his shoes, he lost an important means of mediation, defence, and adaptability for everyday life. However, he was not as frightened as he was confused.

Plasticity is the main feature that distinguishes the element 'earth', as Bachelard observes: 'In effect, as opposed to the other three elements, the earth's primary characteristic is resistance . . . Our way of imagining this material tends to see primal matter, the *prima materies*, in the mixture' (Bachelard 1948b: 10–11). The images in the following dream seem to refer to this mouldable mixture:

> I find myself and the other group members 'dunking' up to our waists in a slimy pond. We play at moulding mud bodies, throwing mud on top of each other, reshaping our bodies with mud, and changing and re-changing our profiles and features. We seem to be having a great deal of fun, even if we are mucked up from head to toe.

This dream highlights the ludic aspect of group work. Here the clay of the 'psychic substance', as Hillman terms it, softens edges, adapts shapes, and changes shapes. A person goes to the group in order to mould and let him or herself be remoulded by his own and the others' psychic substances (Hillman 1979: 152).

As well as this, people who go into a psychodrama group or psychoanalysis often imagine that this will make them more flexible with themselves and the world. The hard edges and angles in the group often become the grounds for conflict and friction. As psychic contents are elaborated, they are replaced by softer lines, flexibility, and malleability. Clay replaces stone as the raw material, even though both are expressions of the same earth element. Clay is thus the first substance on which an alchemical process of transformation is performed. Bachelard and Hillman maintain that psychic substance is characterized by the plasticity and mouldability of clay. Bachelard speaks of dreams as if their shapes originated in the plasticity of the imagination, an imaginative raw material something like dough, clay, or molten metal (Bachelard 1948b: 74ff.). Seconding Bachelard's reflections, Hillman affirms that the essence and nature of dreams can best be defined as a psychic substance characterized by plasticity (Hillman 1979: 152ff.).

No reflection on the element earth and its symbolic value can leave out the earth's most humble aspect – faeces. Although this topic is strictly personal and embarrassing, it recurs rather often in dreams related to psychoanalysis. Faeces represent people's material production, the first thing that is given back to the earth daily. They are the tangible manifestation of people's belonging to the earth. They also suggest the idea of something that is very personal, that continuously reshapes itself, and that one can rid oneself of only for a short time. Hence faeces can be thought of as linked to some irreducible aspects of the unconscious. In the group's collective imagination, faeces make up the raw material that is often brought into the group to be refined and transformed into philosopher's gold by means of alchemical compounds. For this reason it is considered a good sign to have a dream of managing to defecate in the group, getting rid of one's own excrement, and having it all be accepted. It leads to an immediate sense of relief and allows a person to begin the alchemical work of transformation. The group and its leaders are entrusted with the work of reconversion from this raw material. Here is how this theme emerges in one group member's dream.

> I have to go to the second meeting of the psychodrama group, which is being held in A.'s house. I come accompanied by the woman whose house it was into a big room where there is a circle made up of many toilet bowls alternating with luxuriant apartment plants. I have a certain feeling of embarrassment and I wonder if all the stuff flushed down drains into the same point in the centre.

On the other hand, the theme of transformation into precious material is expressed in this part of a dream retold by a woman group member some time after she first joined the group: 'I realize that I have defecated a little jade Buddha.'

WATER

Like earth, water is an element that has been considered feminine. In groups and dreams of groups, water is often related to various phenomena – the feelings, the emotions dissolving into the tears, the ability to melt, the emergence of reflected images that take shape and dissolve, humidity, and plasticity. Tears often mark the emotional entrance into the group, especially for women, who feel more at home with the liquid element of water. Crying is often connected with the fantasy of letting oneself flow into a river of tears, dissolving and turning into a little lake, drowning in one's own tears, and losing one's own consistency. This consistency is like a material that is resistant but then softens and dissolves while crying marks the breakdown of psychic resistance.

Thus a person who weeps and offers his or her own emotions to the group is more exposed and defenceless, but is more approachable. This can happen as long as the crying is neither an expression of rage and isolation nor a kind of liquefaction inside a beetle-like armour plating or exoskeleton. A crying person is more open to contact and to getting in tune with other group members and therapists. They all can feel united in the common feeling of taking in the suffering. This allows them to gather in that part of the suffering that is not just individual.

It often happens in the world of the unconscious that earth and water stand in relation to each other, as in this dream that a group member related shortly after her entrance into the group.

> I find myself with some other people. We have to undertake a sea voyage in a big boat, which maybe we have just built ourselves. The sea is far away. Yet I know that to reach it we have to go down a rough road that passes through the mountains and is bristling with difficulties. Even though it may be tiring, I know that there is a shortcut. When we finally arrive, I feel a great sense of relief and come face to face with the open sea.

The dreamer was a young woman psychiatrist at the beginning of her own analytic experience in group and individual therapy. Until then she had lived very much in the dimension of the earth. As she related in her associations, she felt that she had directed all her energy towards putting together and perfecting her practical life. She had studied medicine and her field of specialization assiduously. By then she had become an able and efficient professional, an expert in organizing effective community health programmes for the outpatient clinic where she was working. This was what her life 'on the earth' was like.

In any case, she was always on the run. The goals she had set before had made her turn a rather deaf ear towards the cries that came out to her from her soul's watery element. She had graduated from a university, completed her specialized studies, taken a job as an assistant in the heath service, and had been promoted to a higher level – all with relentless timing. Her soul struck back at her. It made her anxious to the point of her having palpitations that she associated with an annoying hypertension.

After she made her associations about the dream and participated in the enactment of the dream one session later, it became clear what she had been expecting the group to do for her. She had been hoping that they would allow her to get in touch with the element of water so that she could finally face 'the open seas' without risking shipwreck or dissolution. She connected water with the world of sentiments and emotions. Water represented the pain involved in opening herself up to feelings and reviewing her life history and a personal life that was rife with repressed sorrows that had not been dealt with. She specifically associated the open-sea water with something else she had expected from the group – a sort of exploration of the 'universe beyond the Columns of Hercules'. Yet she realized that the sea might have been near, but that she had to reach it by going down a hard and trouble-ridden road and by tiringly dragging her own boat on her shoulders with the help of the group.

In the following session she connected the water of sentiment with the possibility of weeping in the group, which had been denied her until that moment. A short time later, intense feelings and emotions began to arise in her both in the psychodrama encounters and in individual therapy. These feelings were accompanied by many tears, no longer repressed, and by images of unspecified waters that made their appearance in her dreams. She found that she was newly able to get in touch with those parts of herself that were in pain and that she could again be moved. Shortly after, she dreamed a dream in which the element water re-appeared and was associated with authenticity and freshness:

> I find myself in a house with different rooms. There are D., N., and A., who are maybe working on a big pile of clay in the middle of the room. They seem to be very involved in the work they are doing. I am attracted by a room on the side with greenish walls that seems empty. On entering I feel overrun by a deeply pleasant feeling. I then realize that very fresh spring water is running down the walls of the room and I am taking in airiness and lightness.

This characteristic of the element of water has been described by Bachelard in this way: 'The song of the stream is fresh and clear too . . . This laughter and this babbling are, it seems, the childhood language of nature. Infant nature is speaking in the brooks' (Bachelard 1987: 47).

When the element water appears in the group's dreams, it often means that the ego is beginning to ease its grip, to loosen up, and to soften in order to make room for the element of the anima, its language, and its chances of expressing itself. Hillman writes of dreams: 'Entering the waters relaxes one's hold on things and lets go of where one has been stuck' (Hillman 1979: 152). The dream above was followed by the dreamer working out her problems in harmonizing the earth-bound side of her life, which was very dominant, with her water side. This was something that became the focus of her psychoanalysis for some time. For her the earth meant the everyday world, living with her feet on the ground, and her practical and professional life, where she was doing quite well, even though she had been sticking to rather rigid life styles and roles. For her the world of water meant abandoning herself to her feelings, involving herself emotionally, letting herself be touched, and potentially changing and transforming herself. All this strongly attracted – and scared – her. The fear that she connected with the world of sentiments was the fear that she would lose her usual points of reference, change, and undermine her values in a way she could not control. In short, she was afraid she would lose her identity. When all this came out in individual and group analysis, she was still able to transform herself despite the pain it involved. She could be led to free up the energy and creative potential that she had risked leaving forever 'buried under a kind of too-heavy earth' (as she put it). Not so long afterwards she started feeling as if she wanted to become pregnant – and she did. Needless to say, her life changed. Heraclitus says: 'It is delight, or rather death, to souls to become wet' (Heraclitus 1969: fragment 77; Hillman 1979: 151).

Jung also draws the theme of dissolution – i.e. the 'death of the souls' by water – from the *Rosarium Philosophorum* (Jung *CW* 16; Hillman 1979: 151). Hillman connects Heraclitus's observations on water and death with the well-known alchemical motto, 'perform no operation until all has become water' (Hillman 1979: 153). If we apply this metaphor to psychology, it follows that the *opus* begins with death and that it takes on all the characteristics of an alchemical trans-formation. When an image in a dream is 'wet', it means that the image is beginning to dissolve, is being made more psychic, and hence is becoming more open to transformation. As Hillman puts it, dissolving thus prevents us from being involved in 'fixations in literalized concerns'. Dissolving allows a person to disintegrate 'a kind of too-heavy earth' and turn it into a mouldable element. Since the soul is connected with the liquid element, it needs to flow, filter, and transform itself. All these are the images used to express what is done in the conscious ego.

This process occurs in psychodrama groups. As in analysis, the work begins with the dissolving of the earth and the softening of the 'fixations in literalized concerns'. Psychodrama produces a steady streaming out from earthly concerns and into dreams and enactments that allow the soul to move and the 'psychic material' to flow. At the same time, psychodrama works in the opposite direction. It creates a new earth that stops the flow, an earth defined by the concrete reality of the group and its participants.

Hillman further refers to the traditional association between water and the soul as emotion, feeling, and affect. He distinguishes between a more superficial 'ego-soul', linked to the ego, and a deeper 'image-soul'. The ego-soul corresponds to the surface waters subject to emotional storms that may dissolve it. The image-soul corresponds to the waters of the abysmal depths and the pleasure of being dissolved. 'So, the image-soul's delight is the ego-soul's dread' (Hillman 1979: 152). This is the reason why the analyst-interpreters of dreams who stop at the first image of the ego-soul speak of the risk the dreamer runs of being overwhelmed by the uncon-scious in an emotional psychosis and sunk by the unconscious itself.

The encounter with the ego-soul and, later, with the image-soul in their watery manifestations is illustrated in the following dream.

> I find myself with C. on a beach that is down from a rocky ridge. From a sharp noise like thunder, I understand that the rock is falling and the only way out is to swim across the arm of the sea that I have in front of me. The rocks collapsing into the water stir up whirling, violent waves. Meanwhile, A. and I are swim-ming, tiring ourselves out and risking drowning. When I hit the current I lose my glasses and I turn around to ask A. for help, but I see that she can't help me, because she is struggling against the swells for her very survival. Yet we manage to get to safety up on a new beach on the other side of the arm of the

sea that is not so wide. Starting there, I will cross another city to reach the shores
of the open sea. Here monk seals live. They are wearing white headgear, tied
kerchief-style, under their chins. But maybe what strikes and fascinates me is
the image of the open sea and its calm.

When dealing with stormy waters, Bachelard writes that an onlooker who observes
an extraordinary storm (or experiences one, as in this dream) may find that he is
in an extraordinary psychological state or very shaken emotionally: 'So there exists
an "extraordinary" correspondence between the universe and man, an inner, intimate, substantial communication. The correspondences interweave in rare and
solemn moments' (Bachelard 1987: 232). Here in the first image of the stormy
water in this dream, the dreamer risks drowning by identifying herself with the
ego-soul. This image yields to an encounter with and fascination for the deeper
aspects of the soul represented by the open sea and by its calm.

The other associations with the dreamer's personal life involve her then stormy
affective and emotional world, something that the presence of A. prompted. A. was
a friend and fellow group member who had gone through similar experiences. The
open sea in its vastness and feelings of endless horizons was instead associated with
the image of the monk seals. These feelings can be traced back to the solitary nature
of the inner search that the dreamer was conducting on her individuative path.

On the one hand, the open sea's vastness may upset the ego-soul, which is afraid
of losing its identity when it touches the liquid element. On the other hand, the
open sea arouses an intense attraction for the deeper aspects of the soul. The storm
that was caused by the falling rocks hits an arm of the sea between a beach and
a piece of land beyond that. Beyond this land and towards the open sea, the great
water, just like deep water, reflects its own calm and impassability. This calm is
like that of the 'great white light' of the *Tibetan Book of the Dead*, a light arrived
at only after passing through the terrifying images of the *Bardo* (Lauf 1992: 103ff.;
Jung *CW* 11: para. 831–58).

The seductive and bewitching allure of the waters comes both from their potential
for wealth and the disquieting risk they hold out of dissolution and death. Dreams,
legends, and folklore often express this ambiguity in the image of a seemingly
human creature. Myths attribute god-like features to such a creature. According to
Bachelard, a being that emerges from the water is like a reflection that materializes
little by little. It is 'image before it is being . . . desire before it is image'. Water is
the element specifically associated with fantasizing and with the ceaseless flowing
of reflected images. The features of the Great Goddess can be identified in the
goddesses of the waters and rivers in Iran and of the seas in the pre-Hellenic and
Greek world, according to Eliade (Eliade 1989: 15).

A myriad of figures from folklore, legends, and fairy tales reveal their aquatic
origins. These figures show both sides of the water-unconscious. They are the guard-
ians of endless treasures and wealth as well as harbingers of danger and the desire
for dissolution. These figures are almost always connected with the chance of
becoming wealthy while risking death. Their features are exemplified in the *rusalkas*

of Russian fairy tales (Warner 1995: 28). These are like the Rhine maidens who guard the river treasures and the magic ring and bring death and misadventures with them. They live in crystal palaces on lake bottoms and often have fish tails like mermaids. They have the power to charm and bewitch humans with their seductive voices, beauty, and proffered gifts. Most of the victims are dragged into the water, drowned, or taken prisoner. They have a demonic character that can be defended against by a sign of the cross. One of the characteristics of the *rusalkas* is that they can live outside the water only as long as they are wet or humid. Dryness makes their souls die. Popular legends say that they have an enchanted comb that can make water appear whenever and wherever they want. Hence it may be said that their presence as soul figures in inner images preserves a too solar and too rational spirit from dryness and aridity. Further, the legends say that *rusalkas* climb on to the river and lake banks in the glimmer of full-moon nights. In the same way, inner images emerge and let themselves be glimpsed in the light of the consciousness only in twilight states when the rational consciousness winds down and when 'the lowering of the mental level' (as Pierre Janet termed it) prevails (Janet 1925).

A common figure in Bohemian and Moravian folklore is the *vodnik* – a little man of the waters and dweller of rivers, lakes, waterfalls, and ponds (Ripellino 1981: 6ff.). He comes out of the water in many ways, especially in the form of a kind of open-market shopkeeper wearing an emerald-green frock coat and coral-coloured headgear and sporting aquatic plants intermingled with his hair. Like his *rusalka* neighbours, he can stay on dry land only as long as the left tail of his frock coat keeps on dripping water. When he stops by at fairs and markets, he brings riches to the vendors, who sell him pieces of lace and sequins. Other legends describe him as someone who bewitches people by showing off multicoloured ribbons, little mirrors, combs and pieces of coral, which are really pieces of lake seaweed. He hooks and drags away unlucky swimmers, suicides, and imprudent girls into the abyss and then imprisons the souls of the victims under overturned pots and little silver pans that lie on the river bottom.

Although not necessarily meeting along Central European river banks, psycho-drama groups may also sometimes cause the 'mental level' to 'lower' and 'twilight states' to 'arise' while participants are recounting or enacting their dreams. The group clears the way for these aquatically derived images to emerge, images that sometimes appear in dreams and are then enacted. In these dream enactments the role of the figure emerging from the water may tend to be assigned to one of the two group leaders, as in this example:

> I find myself along a rocky bayside beach that ends with a little fortified city that could be Otranto. On my right there is the entrance to a monastery. I observe its cloister, which has a lazar house inside. The sun is low on the horizon. It could be sunup, but it also could be sundown. The former zookeeper emerges from the water, wet and encrusted with seaweed and shells. I know that we have something important to do together, maybe in the lazar house, and that the job that is waiting for us will be long and hard.

After this dream was enacted, the protagonist connected the image of the cloister and monastery with her search for inner harmony. She associated these buildings with her fascination for the cloister of Monreale in Sicily. She said that she recognized herself in the lazar house and that it took her back to Benares, where she had seen old, emaciated pilgrims waiting to give their bodies up to the water of the sacred Ganges and placing their trust in the possibility of rebirth and regeneration. She also connected the town of Otranto with rebirth and recounted a local legend there in which a sort of immortality was achieved through people denying everything for their faith.

When she played the role of the ex-zookeeper emerging from the water, she said she felt a profound sorrow well up in her because she realized that she was witnessing a world that was in danger of being forgotten and disappearing. She also felt that she – as the zookeeper – was carrying an important message. She had been struck with the real zookeeper's ease with tame and wild animals, his ability to play with them, and their readiness to be guided by him. She had always remained fascinated by this in some way. On the other hand, she had felt that the zookeeper was very introverted, shy, and withdrawn with the visitors to the zoo. She imagined that he had gained a profound skill in relating to the animal world but that he had some problems relating to humans. When considering herself, she felt she was lacking both with animals and humans. Furthermore, her city's zoo had recently been closed and she had found herself worrying about what would become of the ex-zookeeper.

The dream seemed to hold out to her something important 'to do together' with him. Her unconscious had suggested that she work with an internal image of someone who came out of the water and into the conscious world, someone who was able to relate easily with the world of the instincts. This potential was in danger of not being used (as in the closure of the zoo) or of turning bad (as in the zookeeper's alleged problem with relating with humans). She seemingly needed to work on her instinctual side to enable herself to regenerate and get closer to the inner balance she had been seeking. This dream is just one of the many regarding water treated here and in the section on subterranean water in the voyage to the underworld.

AIR

Air has come to stand for the ability to cleave, divide, cut and see clearly. Like fire, it has been associated with masculine characteristics. To understand through the element of air means to understand through the intellect, metaphysical speculation, and the spirit. In psychodrama groups and dreams about groups, the element air can be linked to the life of the intellect, to the understanding of metaphysical truths, and to the rational ability to see the real world clearly. Air may also represent the emergence of aspirations towards a spiritual life and towards an approach to deeper truths. Air is often associated with the images of flight or wings.

Flight is a characteristic that mythical biographies attribute to divine messengers, chosen people and prophets. In this vein, Eliade relates that ancient Indian texts state 'intelligence (*manas*) is the swiftest of birds' and 'he who understands has wings' (Eliade 1967: 105ff.). Flight and ascension to heaven are themes that appear in countless Oriental legends of magic. There are many stories of kidnappings and apotheoses in China, where Taoist priests are termed 'feathered sages' or 'feathered guests'. Taoist priests, as well as alchemists, were said to have to power to levitate in the air. Feathers and bird images may often point to the ability to 'fly into the world beyond' and are hence among the most frequent symbols of shamanic flight.

Celestial flight is a phenomenon characteristic of wizards, sages, and mystics of all types in a variety of cultural areas. Chinese and Hindu alchemists, yogis, sages, mystics, witches, and shamans learn to fly because they take part in a spiritual status for a time. Sovereigns ascend into heaven when they become divine after their deaths. Instead, shamans do not take on divine attributes, but return to earth after their ecstasies. This is their particularity. The image of flight thus represents the ability of certain privileged individuals to give up their bodies temporarily and travel in spirit in cosmic regions, as Eliade points out. The celestial voyage of the shaman is such a flight. Sometimes its aim is to participate in collective religious rituals, such as seeking out the soul of a sick person kidnapped by demons or guiding the soul of a dead person into the other world. Sometimes its aim is to respond to the shaman's own spiritual needs. Something similar happens in initiation rituals that precede death and rebirth when the novice's soul temporarily abandons his or her body and reaches places in heaven or hell that cannot be reached by the living. It is along flight paths like these that the human condition is overcome, at least temporarily.

Psychodrama group work, like individual therapy, may often reawaken fantasies about entering 'another' world of clarity, profound truth, and wisdom, something similar to the cosmic world of pure spirit that shamans, alchemists, priests, and saints enter. The theme of the initiation into flight and shamanic apprenticeship seems evident in the following dream, even if it is handled with a touch of irony by a woman who had finished several years of basic psychodrama and was beginning a psychodrama training group.

> I am walking alone along a deserted street in my home town. It is the main street and it is clear to me that my walk will take me 'beyond the corks'. I keep on the street until I go beyond the city limits and I find myself in a kind of mountainous desert, maybe some area in Mexico. Here there is a man with rudimentary wings – homemade out of bird feathers. He is making a great effort to lift himself up in flight, running up and down to build up momentum. His attempts are extremely rough. They seem more like the flapping around of a barnyard bird than the noble flight of an eagle towards unexplored heights. In any case I know that he will get better. I feel that that flight is about me, as is his aspiration to lift himself from the earth. In his efforts I recognize the

limits on being human and feel both tenderness and tolerance. I recognize how rich and deep was the vital energy that led him to try. This is the dignity I recognize.

The protagonist associated her dream with her condition as novice shaman, something that she called herself with some irony when she talked about her entering the training group. She assigned the role of the figure who tried to fly to the group leader and recognized his skills in trying to fly. She said the landscape reminded her of the shamans from Carlos Castaneda's books, which she had recently read. These shamans did not actually fly, but were able to project themselves and their students towards the infinite; and this was something that fascinated her.

She said the corks she talked about at the beginning of the dream represented a little shop right at the edge of her home town that sold just this kind of merchandise. Her father went there often when she was still a little girl as a point of reference and destination for his solitary walks, presumably absorbed in thought and reflection. Like her father, the dreamer loved solitary walks and trips. She also loved them very much later on in her life even though she tended more than her father – a rather rational man – to live in her imagination. The cork shop and the area on the outskirts of her home town often appeared in her dreams and revealed surprising corners, mysterious unknown neighbourhoods and little shops with the strangest objects. (This was almost a recurring dream.) Here in the dream she had the clear impression of directing herself 'beyond'.

On the individual level, the ability to fly seems linked to a person's rediscovery of their own flying element inside – i.e. the soul or thin body. This does not contain anything material and so gives a person the chance to hover in the sky and move at will. The human imagination expresses this spiritual element of the soul in the shapes of butterflies, birds, or flying animals. For example, a butterfly represents the soul in one of William Blake's paintings (Raine 1958: 155). When a soul symbolized in this way appears in a dream hovering in flight, it almost always carries positive feelings and moods and is often accompanied by feelings of well being. This is evident in the following dream.

> I have the image of a cormorant in front of me, which has appeared to me a lot lately. It has a thick choker collar around its neck. I know that this bird is used for fishing in China and the collar is used to prevent the cormorant from swallowing the fishes it catches so that the fishermen can get them. Me too – I feel like that bird. For a while now I've been feeling a constant feeling of choking at my throat. I finally feel that something is changing. The cormorant is moving more easily. The collar is loosening and falls. Finally the bird stretches out towards the heights and lifts itself into flight. He has cardinal red socks. I feel a feeling of intense relief and profound well being emerge in me.

The dreamer associated the choker collar with the deep sense of oppression that she was experiencing in individual and group therapy, where she was feeling that her blocked emotions were choking her and that she was unable to find a way to express herself. When she played the role of the cormorant as aquatic bird, she recognized the two possibilities it had – to move in the water (like some content from the unconscious that has found its space in the liquid element of the feelings) and to fly up in the sky (like some content involving a spiritual quest). She associated the cardinal red socks with the religious aspects of the dream as a whole. The experience of ascension can be seen as the liberation of a profound aspiration towards spirituality, as Eliade maintains (Eliade 1974: 403). The bird-soul and the butterfly-soul are examples that symbolize this aspiration. Thus spirituality is represented in images as an elevation that is achieved in mystical experience.

The opposite flight trajectory – from the most remote and rarefied parts of the heavens to the earth of bodily life – is illustrated in the following dream.

> I see some winged Pegasuses fly down from a far, far point high in the sky. They near the ground, and land with a certain sweetness and lightness. When they reach the ground, they pee to mark off their territory.

As opposed to the last dream, this dream seems to show the flying element – understood as intellectual expression or approach – transform itself into flesh and blood. This is the association that the protagonist made after the enactment. When she played the role of a Pegasus, she felt that she was going through a transformation that was giving her more bodily and more material characteristics. Even though Pegasuses have wings, they are still horses with all the symbolic implications that go along with that. When they landed on earth and put their hoofs on the ground, they gave themselves up to a more physical existence. In fact, they did one of the most common animal-like things they could – 'pee'. Urinating not only satisfies a physiological need but also serves as a way of marking territory in the animal world. The protagonist associated this urination with the need she felt to make a deeper contact with her more instinctual side. It was as if the contents of the unconscious that had been projected on to a more ethereal and rarefied dimension of thought and emotion felt the need to become flesh and went on to mark out a new existential space and take shape within it. The symbolism of the Pegasus is treated extensively by Erich Neumann in his *History of the Origins of Consciousness*.

> a winged horse, Pegasus, sprang from the decapitated trunk of the Gorgon. The horse belongs to the chthonic-phallic world . . . What the winged horse symbolizes is the freeing of libido from the Great Mother and its soaring flight, in other words, its spiritualization.
>
> (Neumann 1993: 217–18)

Pegasus thus unites the spirituality of a bird with the horse-like character of the Gorgon in one body as a symbol of the stormy and instinctual nature of the unconscious. In fact, the spring that is the source of the Muses, Hippocrene, sprang up from the soil overturned by Pegasus's hoof print.

There are other occasions in which dreamers themselves take flight with the help of a magic instrument, as in this dream.

> I find myself in the psychodrama room. I see the heads and busts of the group members around me. They look like Hellenic marble statues. W. and M., the group leaders, arrive on a magic carpet. They enter through the window and take me away with them. I feel very happy. A gigantic full moon is shining in the sky in front of us.

This dream was recounted and then enacted by a woman who was no longer young and who had not been spared some of the hardest knocks of life. She had brought extremely painful experiences to earlier group sessions having to do with her loneliness, her feelings of abandonment, her seeing the years of her life pass by inexorably, and her increasing weight gain related to serious health problems that seemed to petrify her existence. Nevertheless, what was striking about her was the fresh little-girl-like way of looking that seemed to well up from her bright blue eyes, wide open to the world around her. This was even more striking than the intense sense of suffering that her massive body and weathered face expressed. Her eyes seemed to reflect a kind of unconscious resource that allowed her from time to time to achieve the lightness and elevation that her dream expressed.

The flying carpet of Middle Eastern tales and legends is something that allows a person to ascend and reach an intermediate space from which he can look down from above, i.e. see the world and his own human condition with some detachment. For this reason the fairy-tale carpet is often flying and so fast-moving that it allows the hero to reach the far-away world – the kingdom of gold – and then to return home – his own centre – after he has freed the princess.

While the protagonist was playing the role of herself in the enactment, she felt a keen sense of relief when invited to step on to the carpet. As she said, 'This is the first time in a long time that someone has taken care of me.' She was liberated, at least for a time, of being responsible for other people and meeting their needs, something that oppressed her in her daily life. Hence she could feel like a little girl again and rediscover the dimension of play and stories. After she exchanged roles with W., the woman group leader in the dream, she had the feeling that she had rediscovered the more solid part of herself that allowed her to 'look at herself from above' with more detachment. Every part of her life seemed to be more tolerable when looked at from on high. She said the flying carpet reminded her of the Muslim 'prayer mats' that she had heard about on a tour of the Middle East. In fact, prayer mats often express the soul's nostalgia for paradise and desire for ascension. Their designs often represent celestial gardens with the image of the tree of life (Cook 1974: 59ff.). The tree, like the carpet, marks a sacred space to be used for ascension. Images of expansion, ascension, and flight – usually taking shape as figures of birds – are often designed beside the tree. The Muslim is said to 'fly' towards sacred space on his prayer mat.

There are times when a dreamer may go through a tiring climb in quest of an ecstatic experience, as in the following dream.

> I am wearing myself out climbing up a ladder inside a building whose floors are unconnected and half-demolished. I have to lift up a trap door to get up from one floor to another. At last I reach the roof, which I get up to by removing the tiles. I get to my feet, hold my arms up to the sky, and I begin to fly.

The protagonist enacted the dream and associated it with a mural she had seen on a dilapidated wall of an old building on Portobello Road in London that had struck her very much. On it figures of naked bodies were climbing up the sky-blue side of the house from the windows up to the roof, where a cardboard cutout of a man stretching his hands out towards the infinite stood out. She remembered that she had thought of climbing a stairway to heaven and that this image touched her deeply for an instant. Only a few moments later she remembered that her critical mind had been quick to censor her quasi-mystical feelings with the eye of reason. It made everything seem to her like just a badly made design on a decaying wall and a cardboard cutout in the heart of a flea market. Her dream had seemed to free up the feelings she had censored before.

The protagonist enacted this second scene of the censored emotions also. She felt that it was connected in some way to her perhaps a bit too idealized aim of looking for a kind of ultimate spiritual truth, a search that spurred her to join the psychodrama group. She had repressed this aim and covered it up with more rational ones, just as she repressed the emotion she had felt when first looking at the mural.

Whereas flight is the expression of transcendence and freedom in the more developed cultures, it is the expression of ecstasy in the more archaic cultures. Ecstatic experience is something that is almost rooted in the human experience of a person becoming aware of his or her place in the cosmos. Hence myths and legends of flight can derive from a real ecstatic experience (the trance of a shaman), a dream creation, or a pure invention of the imagination. According to Eliade, flight represents 'a longing to see the human body behaving like a "spirit", to transmute the corporeal modality of man into a spiritual modality' (Eliade 1967: 107).

In this way being able to fly means no longer sharing in human dimensions and being able to transcend them – i.e. 'being in the spirit'. Thus yogis, alchemists, and Buddhist *arhats* (sages) are said to be able to disappear and pass instantaneously from one point to another in space. They are able to transcend and break through the limits of physical reality. The *arhats* are said to 'break and pass through the roof of the house and rise up into the air', something like what happened in the Portobello Road dream. Eliade assesses this motif in this way:

> on the metaphysical plane it is a case of the abolition of the conditioned world. For the 'house' stands for the Universe; to 'break the roof of the house' means that the *arhat* has transcended the world or risen above it.
>
> (Eliade 1967: 109)

There is another way of reaching the heavens besides flying – crossing a rainbow, that magic bridge between earth and heaven for many peoples, as in the following dream.

> I climb up on a mountain with a fascinating young girl who I don't know. At the summit a splendid panorama opens up on to valleys and snow-covered peaks. I notice some extremely vivid coloured rainbows on the mountains across from us. They form arches of a circle and some of the arches are almost complete circles. The girl tells me that there are twelve of them. I experience a very intense feeling that lasts a few moments and I know that this feeling will disappear quickly like the rainbows in the sky. A little later I have another fleeting vision of rainbows on the drafting table of a designer.

After the enactment the woman non-protagonist who played the role of the unknown girl said that the rainbows reminded her of long-forgotten rainbows that she had discovered by chance in the waters of a fountain. She was able to see these rainbows only fleetingly for a few moments at a certain time of the day when the sun's rays hit the water at a particular angle. The many visitors who admire the grandeur of the fountain rarely notice the rainbows. She associated the fleeting apparition that ended the dream with pieces of infinity, which are sometimes able to flow for brief moments into everyday life. This phenomenon brings us back to Eliade's observation about sacred time: the sacred can manifest itself as a lightning-like opening, a momentary interruption in profane time that allows us to glimpse the 'great time'.

The rainbow again brings up the topic of the *axis mundi*: that there was direct communication between earth and heaven in a kind of 'golden age', that it was interrupted, and that it could be periodically restored through the power of shamans, medicine men, and mythic heroes (Eliade 1974: 133). The rainbow is a bridge between earth and heaven that heroes cross in order to enter the world of the spirits, according to Polynesian, Indonesian, and Japanese myths. The rainbow that appears at the calming of a storm is a symbol of the calming of God and a general expression of harmony and serenity. The seven colours of the rainbow are said to refer to the seven heavens in Indian, Mesopotamian, and Judaic symbolism. Rainbows appear in the iconography of the representations of Buddha, Christian art, and Babylonian ziggurats. Rainbows as bridges towards heaven are often depicted on the drums of shamans, who can ascend to the heavens through the magic of their music.

All the symbolism described above is significant for psychodrama in that psychodrama shares its symbolism with initiation rituals. Rituals should be understood in Eliade's terms as symbolic actions that guide people towards wider and more powerful kinds of reality through the symbolic refoundation of the cosmos. In group members' dreams this ritual passage towards wider and more powerful kinds of reality is often marked by the image of flight related to the element air. The individual group members each have a kind of personal mythologem that exists within the context of the mythologem of the group as a whole. This personal mythologem is able to form by going through the ritual of psychodrama (or the ritual of analysis), which opens the personal mythologem up to the wider and more overdetermined reality of myth itself. This is the way that the mythical nature of psychodrama and analytical work becomes evident: it gives everyday happenings more 'air' – more air to breathe – and enables them to flow into the world of the archetypes. The ritual in psychodramatic work may eventually cause the everyday – the here and now and the then and there – to be examined, to re-acquire its universal characteristics, to pass from some part of the universe into some remote place, and to change its nature from the personal to the more-than-personal.

All this seems to express different features of the same reality, which is manifested in threads that continuously interweave and untangle, like the experiences of the group members who live through the myth of psychodrama. Psychodrama is a myth of the earth because it takes its actions from the actions of protagonists who live and act on the earth; but at the same time it is a myth of the air because it allows the protagonists to distance themselves in flight, to look at themselves from above, and to 'take their wings'. The air may also be considered the intellect, rational understanding, the power of discrimination, and the quest for spirituality that emerge out of the everyday. In fact, the personal mythologem of Moreno (as we have seen) contains the myth of a god who looks down upon the world and re-creates it.

Participants in psychodramatic actions can have the chance to look at themselves from above and to re-create their own cosmos and inner reality from that perspective whenever possible. In psychodrama they can be motivated more or less consciously to summon the wings of intellectual understanding related to thought or the wings of inner quest related to the spirit. They share in the myth of psychodrama and analysis as a myth of searching beyond the borders of what is known, like the myth of Ulysses sailing beyond the Columns of Hercules. However, participants may push this quest too far and thus risk losing contact with the everyday world (as witnessed in the dreams about shoes). If this happens, psychodrama is liable to change everything quickly, to follow unknown rules, to rotate the bases of things slowly and almost imperceptibly like a kaleidoscope, and to change their symmetry. Everything can change into its opposite in a few seconds with the same unpredictability of a dream. Scenes can turn from comic to tragic or from the sublime to the ridiculous as they reveal the *enantiodromia* characteristic of the world of archetypal images (i.e. their tendency to turn into their opposites).

Protagonists may find that they have flown in the rarefied atmosphere of the sublime but that they have crashed down in the middle of some of the meanest aspects of everyday life because the sublime and the everyday may come out of the same matrix. Their myths of Ulysses are thus changed into myths of a handsome and ethereal Icarus who has fallen on a rubbish heap, as testified by the great number of dreams about eagles and other noble flying creatures that have fallen to the ground miserably. Protagonists can use their sadness and sometimes their irony to get themselves back into the human perspective, which perhaps has something of the divine whose vestiges are kept in the reality of the soul.

FIRE

Fire is the last of the four elements to be treated here in connection with its associations with symbolism in mythology, in folklore, and in the dream and analytical work of participants in psychodrama. In Bachelard's work on the elements, he identifies fire with what brings on a quick transformation. It is also what can express the desire to hurry up and 'burn the times' and life itself, thus making regeneration possible. Bachelard writes:

> If all that changes slowly may be explained by life, all that changes quickly may be explained by fire . . . that which has been licked by fire has a different taste in the mouths of men. That which fire has shone upon retains as a result an ineffaceable color. That which fire has caressed, loved, adored, has gained a store of memories and lost its innocence . . . We can distinguish then between many kinds of fire – gentle fire, cunning fire, unruly fire – by characterizing them according to the initial psychology of the desires and passions.
>
> (Bachelard 1964: 7ff., 57, 36)

Following these different patterns, fire can take on different features when participants distribute and play roles in psychodrama. There are those who bring the spark that starts to light the fire. They inject and mobilize energy in the group and help make it circulate. There are those who bring irony and liveliness and those who bring impetuous energy, involvement, and intense and violent emotions. There are others who harbor rancours and then let them loose – rancours that they hide like coals under the ashes until something fires them up again. Finally, there are the vestals and the priests of fire, who conserve its integrity and constancy.

Within the psychodrama group, fire is what shines, brightens, and heats at the centre of the circle. It is energy that circulates, affection that is unlocked, feeling that is shown, and anger that breaks out. Fire is the warming at the home fireplace's steady glow. At the same time, fire is 'burning one's tail feathers' in the dynamics of the group. It is a reflecting on one's own and others' burning by life with the help of the therapists and the other participants. Fire is also a soothing and healing of these burns. Fire is a tempering of oneself in the flames of the emotions. The flame that burns at the centre has been created, lit, and continually fed by the energies of the participants. It is the flame where the altar of sacrifice is found. Here something personal is sometimes brought as an offering or is sacrificed in the fire of a continuous search. Memories, dreams, and fantasies become concretely real in psychodramatic space.

Fire can take the shape of the fulcrum of energy situated at the centre of the room in group members' dreams. This is similar to what we have seen in Chapter 5 on the theme of the *axis mundi* or magic tree. Fire appears like this in the following dream:

> We are seated in a circle around a bonfire in the centre of a room where the psychodrama group is usually held. The fire heats without burning. Once in a

while, someone of us throws a piece of wood into the pile, which burns and shines in unexpected ways. The only light that is shining is that of the flame and the small tongues of fire. I am struck by the fact that the contrast of light and shadow changes continuously and changes the expressions on our faces. A welcoming heat glows out of the centre and we all let ourselves be wrapped up in it.

The fire at the centre and the celebrants in a circle around it recall the mandalic image of harmony and integration that turns up everywhere and in every epoch. It burns in scout camps (as one dreamer associated) and in outposts in the most remote corners of the earth. We find fire in the hearth at the centre of the *yurta* – the tents of the heroic knights who are the protagonists of the *byliny*, the epic tales of medieval Russia – and in the tents in the villages of some Siberian ethnic groups. The fire in the tent is located below the hole left for the smoke to rise out of (Warner 1995: 11). Everything that fire has transformed into flying material forms a column of smoke that passes through the upper opening and disappears in the skies.

Eliade recounts how some ethnic groups, such as the Buryats, celebrate a ritual consisting in walking around the hearth, a kind of *axis mundi*. Eliade also discusses Agni, the Indo-Aryan god from the ancient Vedic era (Eliade 1978: 208). Agni was sacred fire, the lord of the home and the fireplace god. As such, he was able to crush the shadows, to chase demons away, and to protect people from diseases and witchcraft.

Just as the fire at the centre of the group can be the flame that heats and brightens, it can also be the alchemical fire of cooking and transformation, as expressed in the following dream (treated before in relation to the sacred meal).

The psychodrama group is preparing a meal. Everyone is sitting in a circle. At its centre there is a big cauldron boiling over a wood fire. Every once in a while someone gets up, goes near the pot, stirs, checks how cooked the food is, smells, tastes, and adds some ingredient. As it is being stirred, I notice that there is a shoe cooking in the cauldron too.

The fire here is the alchemical fire of transformation that gives the group members the chance to share in its benefits. It is possible to participate together in a transformational process like that effected in the group. Here the work of the fire makes food more digestible through cooking. Hence fire can give the participants the chance to transform their memories, moods, and conflicts and make them easier to assimilate. The group waits for nourishment and the chance for regeneration from the magic cauldron at the centre.

It is true that the hearth fire of the group is often associated with heat, affection, and welcome. However, sometimes this fire can express chaotic and destructive qualities. Aside from the image of the fire at the centre of the hearth as *axis mundi*, there is the fire of anger, passion, and intense emotion that can express the violent and chaotic energies that in-depth group work can reawaken. For this reason participants may feel that there is rising up in them an intense feeling of threat, attack, and bombardment. This is illustrated in the following dream related by a woman at a difficult moment in her group work.

> I find myself crossing wide streets in a city at night, pedalling a strange kind of velocipede [early bicycle]. It is shaped like an old wrought-iron Vespasian, like the ones in fashion at the beginning of the century, and it is mounted on a bicycle. There are people who are throwing grenades from the sides of the streets. The street is full of holes and explosions. I am very afraid, but I also have the feeling that I have to continue and learn to live with the explosions without letting myself be intimidated and without stopping.

The dreamer associated the grenade throwers with group members or at least the inner parts of them that she felt threatened by, but she did not manage to identify what those parts were. The Vespasian (an oval-shaped enclosed public urinal, a convenience instituted by Emperor Vespasian himself) seemed to be an image of the psychodrama group seen as a place where a participant could free 'the excrement of the soul'. However, things were not as simple as that, as the dream illustrated.

This following dream expresses the same topic as experienced by a different dreamer: 'N. is in front of me. He looks at me with a provocative look, lights a cigarette, and swallows it.' In the enactment and in his associations, the protagonist identified N. (a psychiatric patient) as part of himself. The protagonist had often brought 'scorching' contents to the group that had to do with his personal life and the group itself, but these were quickly 'swallowed' without being worked out. After this dream, however, he began to work these things out. As we see, what a participant often asks is that the group transform his destructive, chaotic, threatening, and senseless energies in an alchemical fire. He wants this fire to light up a direction for him and to become an *axis mundi*, a starting point for the reconstruction of his inner cosmos.

The transformation of destructive energy into alchemical fire is expressed in this dream.

> I find myself with my cousin in the country house where I grew up. I feel something very threatening in the air. I see a red incandescent ball in the window of a half-basement. I realize that they are conducting an experiment with nuclear fusion. We run away in terror. A little ahead, not very far way, I see a light blue flame in the window of a house. Next to it there is my father who is cooking. The scene brings me back to my childhood, and I feel with relief that there is no more nuclear danger.

The protagonist's relief in the dream corresponds to the transformation of destructive energy into the beneficial energy associated with the light-blue methane flame for cooking food. The nuclear energy that was feared to explode was transformed into a domestic fire that had the benefit of fire for cooking. Bachelard writes the following about fire:

> Among all phenomena, it is really the only one to which there can be so definitely attributed the opposing values of good and evil. It shines in Paradise. It burns in Hell. It is gentleness and torture. It is cookery and it is apocalypse.
> (Bachelard 1964: 7)

In consequence of this, it is not surprising that the ancient Vedic god Agni is represented with two heads in iconography (Moretta 1982: 48). Agni played a fundamentally important role in Vedic religion, and the two heads probably represented his double nature. Agni was simultaneously the emblem of light on earth and fire in hell. His benign nature was expressed in the creative, life-giving fire. At the same time, Agni was dryness, death, and destruction. As divinity, Agni contained the bi-polarity of the archetype. In *Symbols of Transformation* Jung writes:

> If one worships God, sun, or fire, . . . one is worshipping intensity or power, in other words, the phenomenon of psychic energy as such, libido. . . . To anyone who understands libido merely as the psychic energy over which he has conscious control, the religious relationship, as we have defined it, is bound to appear as a ridiculous game of hide-and-seek with oneself. But it is rather a question of the energy which belongs the archetype, to the unconscious, and which is therefore not his to dispose of. . . . Religious regression makes use of the parental imago, but only as a symbol – that is to say, it clothes the archetype in the image of the parents, just as it bodies forth the archetype's energy by making use of sensuous ideas like fire, light, heat, fecundity, generative power, and so on. In mysticism the inwardly perceived vision of the Divine is nothing but sun or light, and is rarely, if ever, personified.
> (Jung *CW* 5: para. 128, 130, 138)

Through the divinity, therefore, people venerate the energy of the archetype or the psychic force that is active in it. In this way, the image of the flame or the sun, in its aspect as producer of warmth and transformation, is a manifestation of the archetype that becomes an emblem of the divinity. Gold, too, corresponds to fire and the sun. It is the alchemical symbol of an incorruptible substance that has the characteristics of divinity itself. In fairy tales, gold is often found in the kingdom of the sun. The search for, discovery, and conquest of golden objects often makes up the ultimate goal of the hero and heroine.

As Maria Louise von Franz has convincingly demonstrated, gold represents the realization of the Self on the psychological level. This can be compared to the rediscovery of one's own fire and inner energy (Franz 1983: 21ff., 1990: 40ff., 1996: 26, 82–83). The representation of psychic energy, which belongs to the inner part of an individual, is often expressed through images of fire and light. This is exemplified in the flame of the Holy Ghost, the halos of the saints, and the shining lotuses that represent the yogic *chakra*.

In many initiation rites, the novice is elevated to a divine condition. He or she is made a participant in the divine essence and becomes aware of this participation in himself or herself. This aspect is often depicted in iconography in the form of fire or light. Such is the theme of many initiation rituals, and the theme of the following dream, already discussed in Chapter 2, on psychodramatic space.

> It is evening and I find myself in Piazza S . . . [a square where the room in which the group usually meets is located]. The city is deserted. I realize that other people are coming up to me in the square. There are five of us in all. I recognize other members of the psychodrama group. We arrange ourselves in a circle with the feeling that we are waiting for something. Five balls of fire come down from the sky and fall down at our feet marking off a pentagram.

This dream, with its sort of initiation into a divine or priestly condition, brings to mind Agni and his cult in the light. Significantly, Agni is also the symbol of the great priest in Aryan-Hindu civilization, where the cult of the sacred fire was practised. Agni is the inspirer of the prophetic priests of Vedic civilization (Moretta 1982: 50).

Fire can be the spark that gives energy, life, intellectual understanding, and the intuition of profound truth. It appears as such in this dream (treated before in relation to the underworld and the earth).

> I feel strongly attracted by a cave whose mouth I see. I venture to go into its depths and I make out a stretch of sand on the inside that I had not noticed before. It is glowing weakly. Suddenly I notice that my mother is next to me. She shows me some sparks of fire on the sand. She explains that if you blow on the sparks, they change into fires and materialize into images of warriors.

Here the sparks are hidden in the depths in the 'reign of the mothers'. The real mother is the keeper and guard for these sparks. In the female dreamer's associations (as we have seen before), the mother was an extremely powerful figure. She associated the sparks with her chance to have biological and spiritual life be born from herself and with her finding out some deep truth about life itself connected with sexuality. Here her problem seemed to be tied in with her ability to re-appropriate this potential.

It has been noted that fire symbolism often touches upon sexual themes. On this topic, Bachelard describes an Australian aboriginal legend that tells of men who did not yet have fire and did not know how to produce it and of women who did (Bachelard 1964: 36–37). The women held the hot coals lit inside their vulvas so that the men could not see them. In a South American myth the hero wants to capture fire. He follows a woman, captures her, and forces her to reveal the secret. The woman tries to flee many times. Then, she hits her stomach hard and a ball of fire comes out of her genitals and rolls down on the ground. In general, fire is often stolen in legends and myths. It is frequently a small animal who steals fire from something or someone who is bigger and more powerful. It is often a wren or a robin, a humming bird, a rabbit, a badger, or a fox, whose red tail gives evidence of his theft of fire.

The dream above of the daughter about her mother does not speak directly about stealing fire, but the protagonist related that appropriating maternal fire was one of the most important issues in the dream.

On the one hand, the dreamer associated the sparks with sexuality. On the other hand, she connected them with finding out a very deep truth about life itself. Her mother was the keeper of this secret and it was fundamental for her to appropriate that secret for herself. This is something similar to a condition that Bachelard has reflected on, the so-called 'Prometheus complex'. It is the Oedipus complex as applied to intellectual life – that is, the urge that carries a person incessantly to want to 'know more' than his or her father, mother, or teachers.

As synthesis of opposites, fire is the symbol of sin and evil as well as a symbol of purity and purification. It burns in hell and, at the same time, it purifies and regenerates in the image of the universal judgement. Bachelard writes:

> Fire is *all-purifying* because it suppresses nauseous odors . . . fire separates substances and destroys material impurities. In other words, that which has gone through the ordeal of fire has gained in homogeneity and hence in purity.
>
> (Bachelard 1964: 103–04).

The purifying function of fire is at the centre of the meaning of cremation in Hinduism, where it is thought that only ascetics and babies do not need to be guided to the other world through ritual cremation (Gonda 1960: 130–38). In Aryan-Hindu tradition, Agni is the 'devourer of the flesh', the purifying symbol of the mortal body. His vehicle is the ram, the sacrificial animal (Moretta 1982: 50). Life itself is fire, combustion, and light. Eliade describes Agni in this manner:

> In the Veda, the god Agni supremely represents the sacrality of fire . . . He 'is born' in the sky, from which he descends in the form of lightning, but he is also in water, in wood, in plants. He is further identified with the sun . . . He is the 'messenger' between sky and earth, and it is through him that offerings reach the gods. But Agni is above all the archetype of the priest; he is called the sacrificer or the 'chaplain' (*purohita*).
>
> (Eliade 1978: 208)

As we have already seen, the priests of Agni are often considered seers. The following dream seems to refer to prophecy connected to purification.

> At the centre of a field bordered by a circle of fire, I see an altar and a pyre where commonly used objects are burning. Among them I make out clothes,

books, appliances, shoes, and utensils. Along with all those, there is a kind of sacrificial animal, maybe a ram, that is burning. I know that this is some kind of purification rite. I am struck by the shapes that the smoke has when it goes up.

Bachelard writes:

> Let us consider now the region in which fire is thought to be pure. This region, it seems, is at the extreme limit, at the point of the flame, where color gives way to an almost invisible vibration. Then fire is dematerialized; it loses its reality; it becomes pure spirit.
>
> (Bachelard 1964: 104)

The representations of Shiva-Nataraj often include the magic circle of fire as the expression of destruction, transformation, and renewal. The god dances in a fiery circle holding a tambourine and a flame in his hands. The tambourine relates to the rhythmic keeping of time and its implacable march. The flame relates to an emblem of destruction and transformation. Several Shiva sects interpret the action of the god in the universe as a cosmic dance through which the god expresses his energy. His dance destroys the world and re-creates it at the same time (Gonda 1960: 214–24). What is destroyed tends toward a greater harmony. The circle of fire represents the wheel of the world encircled by the flames of Agni. In as much as this is a mandalic image, it points to the chance for harmony and happiness within the nature of Shiva itself. According to Shivism, Shiva is the creative power that is able to limit itself and maintain what has been created in balanced harmony. In Shiva there is impure energy, which tends towards the horizontal, the immanent, and the search for power. Also, there is pure energy, which is directed vertically on high as a force that yearns towards transcendence. In Shiva these two forces coexist and are balanced. The dance of Shiva represents the *lila*, or play of the god, through which the phenomenal world destroys itself and is re-created. This image is very widespread in southern India, especially in the temple of Chidambaram near Madras. Shiva is represented in his 108 mystical dance positions. According to the *Tantra* these are 108 ways of becoming able to free oneself from Kali-Yuga (the age of darkness).

In the dream cited above, the circle of flame acts differently from the circle of Shiva-Nataraj. The dream circle marks out a sacred space on a field, a horizontal plane of the contingent world. The circle of Shiva expands on high. However, the dream circle tends towards the heights by the very nature of the flames themselves. Here there is also an energy 'of the earth', which expresses itself horizontally and rises towards the sky. This energy can be classified as the first type of energy that tends towards the immanent and the search for power. It manifests itself in group dynamics, in rivalry, and in competition. The second type of energy is that which rises high like a push towards transcendence. It takes shape in the common acknowledgement that one is undertaking an inexorable search for the absolute.

This is something that is manifested in moments of insight. It is made possible through the energy that is let loose by archetypes that manifest themselves from time to time.

Psychodramatic work in groups exhibits a tiring search for equilibrium and harmony between these opposite types of energy, as happens in the dance of Shiva-Nataraj. Eliade says:

> In later philosophical speculations we shall again find some of these primordial images connected with fire, for example in the concept of divine creative play (*lila*) explained on the basis of the 'play' of flames.
>
> (Eliade 1978: 209)

It is the play of the flames and imagination in the group – in its flashes of light and shadows – that creates images that are born and dissolve. There are many kinds of images. They flow. They change. They keep on transforming themselves. In its inexorable flow, all this seems to dissolve and re-create the phenomenal world like the dance of Shiva in its circle of fire. All of this is defined in the appearance and disappearance of memories, enacted scenes, and dream images. The thunderbolts of intuition and the feelings that they awaken are just so many sparks and flashes that light and burn the group and that go out just as quickly.

Chapter 13

The hidden treasure and the white light

When a hero rescues a woman from captivity or wins a treasure – frequent motifs in many myths and fairy tales – what happens is the mythological equivalent of a person's discovery of the reality of his or her soul, as Neumann maintains (Neumann 1993: 196). When myths about creation develop, what happens is that the psyche projects its own primordial creative power on to the cosmos. Hence, in heroic myths and tales, this same creative power of the psyche is being tried out as something human. This something is a part of a human being's personality – the soul.

These motifs often emerge in dreams in the form of an attainment of a goal that enables a person to get hold of mysterious boxes, magic containers, or coffers containing highly personal messages. These objects often come to act like keystones that help the dreamers put together the pieces of some basic problem in their lives. Here is one such example that helps the dreamer understand.

> I enter a house that R., B., and G. [three psychodrama group members] have shown me the way to. I recognize it as my own; but as I go in, I experience an intense feeling of being lost. The house is empty and I get the feeling that only the superstructure is standing while all of the interior still has to be built. In a room there is a table with a box on it. It contains some pebbles, some dry flowers, and some seashells. It is the same box that I had hid very well from prying eyes when I was little. After that, I never found it again. There is also a little marzipan house with a puppet next to it. This puppet may look like me, but it really is an hourglass.

In the dream the psychodrama group served to point the way inside the house. In the enactment the protagonist played the role of herself and exchanged roles with R., B., and G. (the companions who showed her the way). As she said, she felt she came to posses the truth in a significant way because she began to fit more solidly into the group environment. In the role of herself she said she experienced an intense feeling of expectation when she got the directions from R., B., and G., as if the presence of the others had mobilized her energies. As the scene progressed, she instead felt loneliness, disorientation and fear as well as curiosity.

It came out clearly that she was going back and forth between two feelings. On the one hand, there was her trust in the group that was linked to the security that her sense of belonging gave her. On the other hand, there were her desire and curiosity that pushed her to go on by herself. These two feelings turned out to be complementary. It seemed to her that the group was showing her something and pushing her towards a goal that was paradoxically something very personal. Hence the group's hidden treasure seemed to be her own individuality.

The goal of her dream quest was her connection with her past. At the time of the dream she had been going through profound changes and transformations in her life. She was finding it very hard to find continuity in herself. She was beginning to realize that she deeply needed a pattern or superstructure that could give her a sense of shelter and stability. Until then her life had been led as a series of constant and frenetic changes. At that time she had just changed jobs and lovers.

She recognized that the house's superstructure and the solidity it implied – even empty – represented the continuity that she needed. She associated the house's solidity with a certain self-confidence that the group helped her reach. In fact, her dream companions had helped her find her way. On the other hand, the house was only an empty structure that needed heat into order to make life possible. This was tied in with her frustrated desire for maternity. She associated her finding the box with her recovering something that was lost, that was 'hers and hers alone'.

The little marzipan house made her reflect on the fact that she might always have been a bit too hard on herself, that she had denied herself the possibility of 'sweetening up her life'. The hourglass-shaped statuette or puppet made her reflect that time was going by, that she considered herself an 'eternal adolescent', and that she had begun to feel the growing need to relate as an adult among adults.

The dream of another participant, a 45-year old woman, brings up the problem that she had not become a mother and that she subsequently refused to face this issue emotionally.

> Finally I find myself on a path through the fields. I see my father-in-law come towards me with a little coffer. I have the feeling that this is exactly what I had been looking for to give me the key to what is happening to me. When I open it, I see that it contains a pumpkin seed that has been sewn up and a ring with a bezel. The ring opens up and inside I distinctly see an egg-cell. I realize that it is mine and I become aware that I have always kept it jealously for myself imprisoned in a ring.

The protagonist chose the male co-conductor to play the part of the father-in-law. By casting him as her father-in-law, she realized that she expected him to hand her back her creative potential during her analysis. At least, he should make her aware that she was cut off from her creativity. In the dramatization she held the coffer in her hand and opened the bezel of the ring. She commented that this brought into her mind the living image and the intense colour of an egg-cell imprisoned in a double wrapping. She then remembered an embroidery that she made as a little girl in a convent school sewing course. She had wanted to embroider poppies on a linen napkin, but the nuns made her copy 'little pallid, slightly-faded flowers'. Sometimes her life seemed just like that.

She said the stitches in the pumpkin seed also reminded her of the sewing episode. In this light she saw the nuns as that part of her own austere and rigid internal images. Her whole life long, they had been inhibiting her from enjoying pumpkins with their magical transformations or poppies with their bright reds. The dramatization brought her intense suffering and profound sorrow to light. She reflected that she had started to want her group work to help her free her feelings and sensitivity from their prison. Even though she was past the childbearing age, she saw her group work as bearing fruit in the reawakening the creative potential of her feelings.

Finding the treasure in the following dream is related to the theme of a person recovering her energy in the realm of professional skills: 'At the bottom of the wardrobe I finally found a box that I had lost. It is shining. It holds a pair of championship skates that I am proud to show off to the group leaders.' At that time the protagonist was working out her problem of low self-esteem on the job, something that she had long been projecting on to the group and its leaders. When she played the role of herself, she said that the skates in her hand made her feel deeply satisfied. They made her feel like skating. She wanted to show the others how good she was, but what she wanted more was to show this to herself. She associated all of this with the feeling that she again had found her lost energy that was only waiting to be tapped. After she played the role of the group leaders who were shown the 'championship skates', she saw them as some of her own inner qualities that were finally beginning to 'legitimate themselves'. She associated this scene with a professional project that she was very proud of. This was a project that allowed her to reap the benefit of the growth process she had been going through up until then in group and individual work. At the same time, this project guaranteed that she could exploit her creative skills fully and originally. She was also proud that she had had the courage to propose her project at her rather rigid and conformist work place and win its approval.

Other times, finding the treasure may also involve rediscovering something of one's own that was given little importance or even hidden with a certain embarrassment. The treasure in this dream is hidden in household rubbish. This image recalls Hekate's sacralized rubbish, a topic treated before in relation to death in the voyage to the underworld and to be taken up afterwards in the book's conclusion:

> I then understand that the treasure was hidden right in the centre of the room, where the group told me I had hidden the rubbish under the rug. At that time I had seen swarms of cockroaches come out of there and, later, I had seen a fire glowing that heated without burning. There, under the floorboards, I find some gold coins again. They have hardly any commercial value, but have a deep emotional significance for me.

The protagonist was a 40-year-old man with some rather obsessive traits. In the group he had often been pointed out for his way of presenting himself only in a 'formal and well-bred' way that attempted to stifle and hide his shadow. He had been told sarcastically by a woman participant: 'Whenever you bring something into the group, it looks as if you're worried about showing us a house that's always neat and clean. You're always sweeping the dirt under the rug.' He had this dream several months after her comment. Indeed, he was used to presenting his social wrappings, his conformism, and his 'good manners'. Very little or nothing of his emotions or sentiments ever leaked out. These were constantly repressed, hidden, or experienced as weaknesses that he had to be ashamed of. These were the emotions and sentiments that appeared in the image of the rubbish under the rug with its swarms of cockroaches. The protagonist said that this dream made him able to discover the warmth of his emotions in the fire at the centre of the room and the authentic emotional value of his life history in the 'coins of little value that still had a deep significance for me'.

Seeing white light or being surrounded by white light is another way dreams have of expressing that a goal has been reached. Fairy tales express this in terms of heroes discovering treasures, and myths express it in terms of heroes conquering death. White light is perhaps the symbolic representation that an essence is spiritual or that the quality of *mana* has been bestowed on the people manifesting it, as in the following dream.

> I find myself at the day hospital at night in the middle of people who are sleeping. Everything's dark and I feel pretty uneasy. I hear some steps and I see M. come down the stairs. He is wearing a glowing white shirt.

During this period the protagonist was doing her first practical internship as a psychologist in the psychiatric day hospital where the dream was taking place. She was in contact with grave forms of psychosis. Her internship aroused strong, confusing, conflicting emotions in her that she was finding hard to work out.

She associated the night in the dream with her abandonment of rational defences, the time when she could see the 'light in the darkness' and achieve a new form of consciousness. This came in the form of the glowing white shirt worn by the group leader, himself a long-time psychologist among gravely ill psychotic patients at the same centre. This is the reason she had imparted him with the healing force of *mana*. In the role of herself she felt both frightened and attracted by the atmosphere she was moving in, which she associated with the fascinating and deeply disturbing internship she was going through. She noticed she really wanted to have a guide to support her on her path of progress, which she associated with her participation in the psychodrama group. When she played the role of the group leader as he appeared in the dream, she felt that his shirt's brightness came out of his profound experience at work and his long journey in analysis. These gave him the ability to move even in the dark without feeling disoriented. After first feeling confused, the protagonist felt the presence of this guide figure in herself.

Sometimes the white light appears as a pure essence that wraps around reality, transfigures it, and takes it into a spiritualized dimension, as in this dream.

> I am woken up in the middle of the night by an intense white light. It is the light of the night. I then understand that this is a light that has always existed but is impossible to see with the eyes of everyday life. The light shows itself only little by little and only for a very short time. I then remember the feeling that I had already seen it a long time before and I wonder how I could have forgotten that it existed. I look out the window and see that there is a big festive crowd all dressed in white and they are walking in the light. There are faces that I know – relatives, friends, and significant people in my life – mixed in with faces that I don't know at all. I feel the light that unites me with them. I go down and out and I immerse myself in the crowd and let myself be carried along.

After the male protagonist told the dream to the group, a deep silence followed. Finally the group leader asked the participants to enact the part of the dream that involved going out into the street and immersing themselves in the crowd. He asked them to play the scene without words, slow their movements down as much as possible, and let their emotions flow into the atmosphere of the scene. All the group members participated. The dramatization was extremely intense and represented a very meaningful moment in the life of the group, even though it probably took on features very different from those of the dream itself. The experience was such that it could only be conveyed through participation, presence, silence, and gesture. In this context verbal experience seemed to be entirely inadequate to express the intense emotions aroused, except for the words of one participant thanking the protagonist for bringing the dream to the group. The participants were given the freedom to evoke their musings, images, and personal contents, some of which were shared and worked on in later sessions. This scene was the last one enacted in that particular psychodrama session and was again dealt with in the conductor's final observations and made to fit into the context of the whole session.

The vision of the white light is represented in some shamanic initiation rites by the *quamenec*, a mysterious light that the shaman unexpectedly feels as bright fire, according to Eliade (Eliade 1967: 83). This makes him able to see in the dark and to make out things, future events, and secrets that cannot be known by other people. An existence is revealed to the shaman, which, although belonging to the world, is founded on other existential dimensions. The initiatory passage of the *Bardo Thodol*, the Tibetan book of the dead, is analogous. The dying person must know how to identify himself with the great white light that shines beyond the karmic images of human existence (Neumann 1993: 196).

All in all, the 'hidden treasure' can come to stand for what each group member is seeking on his or her individuative path as he or she passes through the psychodrama group. The hidden treasure may stand for a more collective search for meaning. It may represent symbolically a kind of resolution or, better, a presentation of the issue that is then at the centre of each group member's analytic quest. In this way, the treasure can take on different appearances from time to time. The treasure may be an hourglass as a search for stability in change, an egg-cell as a problem with fertility, championship skates as professional success, a white light as the quest for religiousness, and countless other shapes.

Conclusion

What this book has been saying is this. Psychodrama is a ritual. It takes mythical material. This material consists in the mythologems of the individual participants and of the group as a whole. These mythologems – the stories or parts of stories that people tell or imagine or dream or project about themselves or others or things – are not static but continually emerging. Psychodrama takes these mythologems and puts them up against aspects and pieces of real-life experiences. If we think back to Eliade, any ritual sanctifies a profane time and space by transporting them into a mythic time and space. Hence the fact that psychodrama is a ritual implies that it delineates a shelter – a *temenos* – inside which its participants can reconstruct a cosmos from the chaos and the unknown of the images that are emerging from the unconscious.

A ritual is a symbolical action taken in order to found the cosmos once more and guide people on their ways towards finding out and taking in ever broader and ever stronger realities (Eliade 1991: 20). Hence psychodrama allows a participant to make the crossing from the chaos of his or her unconscious into the world-cosmos he or she has inside. Here a participant renovates and refounds his or her own personal myth and that of the group, which cannot remain static but must be subject to the continual transformations that keep these myths from the danger of becoming static and rigid.

These transformations come out of constant exchanges and crossings. Psychodrama participants who experience the scenes they play as flesh and blood protagonists cross over to become characters that belong to the inner realities of each of the participants. The opposite crossing is just as real. Internal images, dream projections, and dream characters cross over to become real people – the participants and conductors – in the same way that the very presence of the participants makes internal images emerge in each individual participant. Each participant's internal images reflect and refract the others' images, strengthen them in turn, unite with them, and sometimes open up new pathways.

Psychodramatic play, role exchange, the reflections and recollections that follow, and the emotions and states of being that are evoked are all factors that lead the group members and the therapists to constantly transform themselves, their points of view, and their own inner worlds. All this leads to a plasticity, suppleness and flexibility that keeps them from becoming rigid. This seems to guarantee a continual unfolding of what Jung defines as the 'transcendent function', which is activated by the individual and the group unconscious – and by its potential to establish a relationship with the conscious (Jung *CW* 8: para. 131–93). In fact, a characteristic of the transcendent function is its ability to put the unconscious and the conscious together so that they are constantly linked and dialectically juxtaposed. The transcendent function avoids falling into the trap of supporting either the unconscious or the conscious unilaterally as if either were the sole factor.

In fact, the unconscious, with its knack for showing up suddenly in the group, enables the group members to focus spontaneously on entirely unexpected elements – as happens in dreams – during the dramatic play. These elements can lead participants to differing perspectives, to new openings, and often to different conceptions of reality and of existence itself. It is of fundamental importance for the group members and therapists themselves to create these possibilities and keep them open.

There is something that may seem surprising, but not for those familiar with the techniques of analytical psychodrama. Infinite numbers of apparently chaotic and steadily changing inner images emerge. Yet, in the midst of this confusion, bit by bit, clear pathways emerge. They stretch out one by one while scenes are unfolding and while dreams are being brought into the group by association. Often the roads that are marked out are completely new for the group members and the therapists themselves. They are like beaten paths that sometimes seem cleared, often seem to disappear into fields, and eventually become identifiable when people follow their trail marks. It may be said that these traced-out courses constitute the mythologem of the group in its incessant transformations.

The same thing happens to the group members on their individuative routes. Sometimes the routes start to look like a well-travelled road where all the members meet each other and then go off one by one into the woods. Sometimes they go alone. Sometimes they go down short stretches of the road with one or more of their fellow travellers. The story lines and the routes intersect with each other and lead to surprise meetings. They may be said to represent the individual mythologems of the psychodrama group members, which are strictly linked to each member's individuative journey. It is here where the other group members meet each other again and again. Each time they meet they have changed and they are surprised at rediscovering the stretches where they have journeyed together. Often the most intense encounters occur at these forks in the road or crossroads. Here the chances for the deepest and most immediate empathy develop, burst forth without warning, and sometimes disappear just as rapidly.

Crossroads are places where it is granted that people can see and listen in many ways at the same time, for these are places sacred to Hekate, the underworld goddess traditionally portrayed with three heads. The encounters in these magical crossroads represent new chances for people to look at themselves in the mirror and find an image that is like their own and yet different at the same time. Hekate also has the power to sanctify domestic rubbish, which is offered to her right at the crossroads. In a certain way, she may have something to do with psychodrama if we keep in mind what Hillman says about her in reference to dreams. In fact, dreams are considered refuse by several authors, including Freud himself, who called them 'day residues' (Hillman 1979: 39).

The main road can perhaps be traced back to the myth of analysis or rather – more to our point – the myth of analytic psychodrama. For better or worse this road is always present in this context even though it often seems impossible to chart. The road should not start to feel like a forced march. It should not be fenced in by barriers or by high walls. It should not open on to dead-end labyrinths whose every angle calls for meticulous inspection. As long as this does not happen, such a road has room for group members and leaders alike as they discover new, unexplored pathways and do not hesitate to recognize the pathways that would involve them.

All of this inevitably makes people constantly come face to face with uncertainty and doubt. In fact, every point of reference turns out to be subject to continual change. Just as in dreams, the road travelled can disappear from one moment to another and this makes it impossible for people to retrace their own steps. Thus it becomes important to feel the analytic and psychodramatic route as a path that winds off to lead to thousands of possible routes or roads. If the traffic is directed one way because the analyst or group leader is afraid to lose his or her way on a maze-like route, the road will break off. In other words, we will not be able to get past ourselves and our pathway will turn out to be a dead-end trap if we have persuaded ourselves that this was the only way possible (Gasca and Gasseau 1991: 33).

All this constantly leads the analyst to question himself or herself further and come face to face with his or her own shadow, which inevitably brings up his or her own human limitations, fallibility and doubts about what he or she is doing. The relationship between the analyst and his or her shadow is something presented again and again. It is made up of precarious balances and constantly renewed imbalances. When a person accepts this contradiction, when he acknowledges that he is running the risk of making mistakes, and when he gives up his conviction that he knows what to do in all circumstances, only then can the shadows brighten (Romano 1975: 65).

It is in this uncertainty that initiation symbolism unfolds. In this passage to 'another' world – an underworld belonging to dreams and the soul – rules and known points of reference seem to lose consistency and value. Here initiation symbolism seems to bring us back to deeper and more meaningful values and references that reach another dimension of existence. It brings us back to what our contemporary culture, with its rational and scientific perspectives, tends to take us away from. Thus what happens in work with the unconscious can ultimately be considered a sort of compensation for the attitude of the collective conscious, which tends to consider death as 'the ultimate pathology of the body' and to negate its characteristics as a transforming experience (Zoja 1985: 4ff.).

In view of this, it is important to remember that societies that consider initiation sacred often consider death in the same way. These considerations have come to be lacking in our contemporary western society. Therefore keeping silence, listening, and waiting in group and analytic work allows and encourages themes related to death, initiation, and the very meaning of existence to flourish again. When rational thought is slowed down, it makes room for a twilight zone that lets images come out of the unconscious. Then again, there emerge the eternal, unresolved questions that the conscious has long resigned itself to being unable to answer. Thus the psyche escapes from the self-criticism of the conscious by re-proposing the multiple and inexhaustible responses of the unconscious that cannot be grasped by the principles of logic. Bachelard comments:

> reverie takes up the same primitive themes time and time again and always operates as it would in primitive minds, and this in spite of the successes of systematic thought and even in face of the findings of scientific experiments ... If we force ourselves – and I think we should – to rediscover the imaginary experiences that we have in the great reign of sleep on the threshold of our effective experiences, we would realize that we have been given the day to verify our experiences of the night in the reign of the imaginary and of reverie ... Psychically, we are created by our reverie – created and limited by our reverie – for it is the reverie which delineates the furthest limits of our mind.
> (Bachelard 1964: 4, 1987: 248, 1964: 110)

Glossary

Anima From the Latin, *anima/ae*. A powerfully symbolic **archetypal image** through which different psychic contents from the **personal** and **collective unconscious** express themselves. Anima is a kind of personification of the feminine principle of eros. Anima is represented in dreams through images of women who often take on the function of spiritual guides in as much as they are related to the deepest levels of the unconscious. In as much as anima is the feminine principle, it reveals itself through the contradictory nature of archetypes as the synthesis of opposites. Anima can be at the same time an angelic and a diabolic figure, an ethereal and a terrestrial one, a virgin and a prostitute. *Rusalkas*, sirens and *melusinas*, whose fish or serpent tails betray their underworld origins, often represent the anima in dream and fairy tales. In the world of the psyche, anima brings sensitivity, intuition, empathy, feeling, and inspiration. On its negative side, anima can bring on weakness, hypersensitivity, indecisiveness, the inability to make a choice, passivity, and moodiness. As an internal image in men, anima represents the unconscious feminine part that complements their male identity and compensates for its conscious aspects. Anima allows perceptions related to unconscious processes to flourish. Anima is relatively autonomous from the ego. As a '**complex**' linked to the world of archetypes, it reveals itself to be endowed with a life of its own. Anima gathers up a composite of psychic functions in itself that are often so significant that they constitute an authentic 'secondary personality'. In as much as anima is an 'inner attitude' that reveals the way people address their inner worlds, it stands in antithesis to the '**persona**', which, on the contrary, reveals people's outer attitudes and adaptation to the external world. In psychodrama anima demonstrates itself through projections on to the female figures in the group that come and go through the **role** playing and dream images.

Animus Just as the anima represents the feminine principle or 'eros' in the form of an **archetypal image**, animus represent the masculine principle or 'logos'. In women it represents the unconscious masculine aspect complementary to the conscious feminine aspect. It reveals itself in dreams in the form of masculine personifications. Similarly in the world of relationships, the masculine principle is often projected on to men. The animus can be the carrier of rationality, opinions, judgements, the need for critical reflection, decisiveness, the ability to choose, and the quest for truth and spiritual values. On its negative side the animus can bring on rigidity, intransigence, and a polemical spirit.

Archetype – archetypal image   The archetype in itself is a sort of 'innate disposition to produce symbols'. Jung compares archetypes in the psychic realm to patterns of instinctual behaviour in animal and human nature. In as much as they are the common heritage of humanity, they seem to belong to a sort of inherited structure of the psyche itself and for this reason they appear at all times and places. Whereas autonomous **complexes** are essentially related to the **personal unconscious**, archetypes – analogous structures – are related to the **collective unconscious**. Like complexes, they are characteristically autonomous of the consciousness and equipped with a charge of energy that is decisively more intense because it comes from the deepest levels of the psyche. When an archetype is activated and appears, it can prove to be so extremely powerful that it can sometimes unhinge the very structure of the psyche if it does not find adequate containment. In psychoses in which the structure of the ego is too weak to withstand the impact of the violent energy released, the archetype can show its full power, completely overrunning the contents of the consciousness, which end up reduced to nothing – at least temporarily. Archetypes are not uniquely related to single individuals but to everything that is human in a wider sense. They can be recognized when they appear by the strong, symbolically laden images that accompany their mobilization of intense emotions. Archetypes are linked with situations that lie at the limits of existence and express themselves in symbolic language. They often appear at crucial turning points of existence along with the multitude of psychic contents that have gravitated towards them. Archetypes appear in dreams, myths, and fables as expressions of the collective unconscious in a way that is both peculiar and accessible through images characterized by '**numinosity**'. In psychodrama an archetype displays itself in proportion to the group's and its individual members' openness towards that particular archetype. When an archetype appears, it is almost always prompted by the presentation of images that take on a strong archetypal power and so are able to set off a strong emotional resonance in the group. As manifestations of the collective unconscious, they constitute the roots of myths, legends, and fables. On the individual level, they appear in dreams and fantasies.

Auxiliary ego   The term 'auxiliary ego' indicates the participants in the group who play the various **roles** in an upcoming scene at the request of the **protagonist**. It is worth noting that the protagonist can opt to have another participant in the group – who acts as an 'auxiliary ego' – play the role of himself or herself. The protagonist expects to hear some significant response from the participant who was chosen. In this way the protagonist has the chance to 'see' himself or herself from the outside – at least in a part of the scene. The group members take on a twofold function. First, they are a 'chorus' who participate and comment on the protagonist's actions and so function as an emotional and affective container. Second, they are a gathering of 'auxiliary egos' who have been called into the scene to make the protagonist's inner world something material and concrete; the world that is represented through their physical and emotional presence.

Compensation   According to Jungian thought, the **libido** exercises a continuing compensation for the contents of consciousness by setting autonomous **complexes** and **archetypes** in motion that spread the opposite **enantiodromic** principle through the unconscious. Consciousness, in fact, tends to orient itself by choosing steadily to go one way only and to discard into the unconscious those contents that hinder its advance. These do not lose their charge of energy, a charge that blends in with the libido of the **collective unconscious** itself, which is directed towards **individuation**. In this way the unconscious constantly tends to act to reclaim its own contents by effecting a kind of homeostatic compensation for the consciousness. In psychodrama a meaningful kind of compensation appears in the spontaneous, steady shifting in scenes between contents from real-life experiences and from the dream world.

Complex   By complex is meant a concourse of feelings, thoughts, emotions, moods, fantasies, images, and, sometimes, somatic symptoms that have come together to revolve around a kind of central nucleus. Complexes escape the control of the conscious ego and behave autonomously from it, as if they were endowed with their own lives. They structure themselves authentic personalities that are partial, secondary, and separate from the ego's will and intentions. Therefore complexes can often set themselves up in antithesis to the consciousness's ability to plan. In various circumstances complexes can influence the functioning of the conscious ego or even substitute themselves for it, especially if they join in with the archetypal values rooted in the deepest levels of the unconscious. The conscious ego may come under the sway – as it were – of the complexes and even be overwhelmed by them. Because of this unique feature of theirs, they have been defined as 'autonomous'. They perform the essential function of channelling the flow of psychic energy towards different fields of interest and plan-making. Further, autonomous complexes essentially function to determine the spontaneous emergence of the thoughts, moods, and emotions that cross our minds. They sometimes unwittingly call on these and so get them to act. Although they may stand as obstacles in the way of the conscious ego's attempts to plan, they have a very dynamic character and so can constitute a powerful stimulant for transformation. In dreams autonomous complexes often appear and interact among each other in the forms of characters that appear as dream images. In this way they offer a varied and richly nuanced portrait of what is stirring in the unconscious at that moment and reveal which way the psychic energy is going. Complexes are most related to the psychic contents linked to the **personal unconscious**.

Conductor   The conductor (or leader) performs a variety of tasks. In fact, he or she is the one who guides the group in its incessant explorations inside the labyrinth of relationships, fantasies, encounters, feelings, emotions, images and memories that come out in psychodrama. At the same time, this is the person who looks for some sort of sense in all these phenomena and aims to give them back their form and set them off in some direction. On this pathway he or she reflects a world, which is at the same time that of the relationships among the **protagonists**/participants and that of the relationships among the figures from their inner worlds who continuously enrich and transform themselves in this way. Formulating hypotheses about how themes may develop, a conductor handles the *direction* of the scenes together with the protagonist and the group. Meanwhile he or she maintains the *analytic and therapeutic function* that will allow him or her to have the awareness and responsibility for what is happening and what he or she is doing at that moment. All this is carried out in the group by going in two directions – towards each of the individual participants and towards the group as a whole. Analytical psychology recognizes four fundamental functions in the individual: intuition, thought, feeling, and sentiment. One could say that conducting a group requires that all these functions be involved at the same time, interact harmoniously, and be balanced. In fact, it is important that a conductor participates, allowing himself or herself to be guided by the *sentiment* and the emotions that are flowing through the protagonist and the participants without becoming overwhelmed, and keeping his or her analytic and therapeutic function intact through *thought*. In the same way it is important that a conductor is able to pick the possible roads to go down *intuitively* and that he or she can at the same time recognize the language of the *feelings* that emerge. Besides constructing the scenes along with the protagonist, the conductor also takes on the function of the '**auxiliary ego**' by prompting the protagonist during the dramatization of the scenes.

Enantiodromia   According to the philosophy of Heraclitus, enantiodromia is the tendency of everything to transform itself into its opposite in the game of becoming. What appears to the conscious has a corresponding opposite principle that spreads through the unconscious. In psychodrama it is possible to work on the enantiodromic principle through **role** playing and role exchange with the antagonist. The movement of the **libido**, understood in the Jungian sense, is always directed towards a continual constellation of and compensation for principles opposed to it.

Great Mother   The Great Mother is one of the archetypal symbols that is most often encountered. In synthesis, she represents all the matriarchal divinities as givers of life, nourishment, and well-being. On her negative side she is also the giver of death, capable of devouring, castrating, and killing. She is connected with the image of mother earth as a primordial force of nature that has the potential to create and at the same time destroy and re-absorb what she has created inside her. The inner image of the biological mother can take on disquieting projections related to the image of the Great Mother. The biological mother may appear in people's dreams and fantasies as the Great Mother. The archetype of the Great Mother with her affective, nourishing and simultaneously enveloping and castrating characteristics is often activated in the imaginations of therapeutic group participants as an image of the group itself.

Group   See **Auxiliary ego**.

Individuation   Generally speaking in Jungian terms, individuation means the realization of the potential innate in each individual. Thus the term is connected with the development of the individual's personality through that individual marking the way his or her own uniqueness is different from collective thought and values. In social relationships the process of individuation assumes that an individual relates to others in his or her own unique way and experiences the values of the group he or she belongs to in a more inner-directed and personal way. In this way group values are not accepted passively are but reclaimed and re-elaborated in a spontaneous way, keeping a certain dose of innovative energy alive. In the broadest sense, individuation guides a person towards the realization of the **Self** as the complete expression of himself or herself as a whole. Individuation also stands in relation to a person's fulfilment of their own human destiny. The function that pushes an individual towards this goal is defined as the 'transcendent function'. During the course of an individual's entire existence, the transcendent function relates the consciousness of the ego to the contents of the unconscious, which manifest themselves through a continual transformation.

Libido   In the broad sense, the libido is understood as psychic energy in relation to the intensity of the psychic process. This term in its Jungian form takes on a broader and less determined meaning than the Freudian libido, which is a kind of biological energy directed towards satisfying instinctual needs. For Jung, libido is a pulse of energy that orients thought processes towards the continuous transformation that is effected through the continuous interaction of autonomous **complexes** and **archetypes** in relationship to the consciousness. The libido tends to be directed towards compensating for the conscious contents reflected in individuals' actions and life choices. The libido directs their thoughts and tends towards effecting a homeostatic equilibrium. Understood on a more global level, the libido spontaneously orients itself over the span of a person's entire existence towards fostering the **individuation** process. It does this through helping individuals express their innate potential to bring out their own uniqueness.

Numinosity   By numinosity is meant a particular affective tonality capable of summoning to itself a great quantity of psychic contents and of raising strong emotions connected with everything that represents the inexpressible, the mysterious, and the terrifying. The 'divine' and what Jung defines as the experience of the **Self** are carriers of these attributes.

Observations   The 'observations' conclude the sessions after the '**sharing**'. When there are two group **conductors** who alternate in leading the sessions, one conducts while the second stays apart in a corner of the group taking notes to be fed back at the end of the session. The observations represent a kind of thread that binds the scenes together and, to a certain extent, represents the development of the group's theme. The observations claim to be neither a detailed description of the session nor an interpretation of what has been happening according to logical and rational interpretative tools. These would risk yielding a reductive reading that would follow the patterns of predetermined analytical models. The observations are simply limited to giving back coincidences, images and connections that are open to more than one reading and reflect the individual participants' different ways of seeing and feeling. The observations act as a stimulus to help each participant rediscover some crucial connections through the feedback, words, or images received from them. Further, the observations give the participants the readings that they feel are most their own without having them jump to conclusions. In this way, the end-of-session observations open new questioning and again foster a steady dialogue between the conscious and the unconscious of the individual participants, of the group as a whole, and of the collective. This is a dialogue that stays at the centre of the analytical journey. When a conductor works alone, he or she presents possibly briefer impressions to the group as a sort of device that ties in the collected work done and gives it back to the participants. This context also gives the group the chance to gather in and again take up the **roles**, feelings, themes and emotions of the **protagonists** and participants that may have been left 'suspended' over the course of the conduction of the group because the session had not developed in a way that gave them the chance to be returned to.

Persona   The persona is a sort of 'social mask' through which individuals relate to the external world with varying degrees of success by trying to adapt and conform to what the 'collective consciousness' or the 'significant others' in their lives expect of them. The word 'persona' comes from the name of the mask that the actors in ancient Greek theatre wore as they played various **roles**. It is therefore a collection of functions that aim to 'adapt' a person's individuality to the outer world. As such, the persona stands in antithesis to the 'shadow' – i.e. what good social adaptation deems inconvenient and so is relegated to the world of the unconscious. Analogously, the persona stands in antithesis to the **anima**, which represents a person's attitude towards his or her inner world. Thus the persona is a kind of suit (as it appears in dreams) that comes in the various styles that circumstances call for. It is a 'calling card' that changes prints and titles according to the environment in which it is shown. Excessive identification with one's own social *habitus* stands in the way of the dialogue with the unconscious and hence of the **individuation** process. It is precisely the task of analytical work to remove these obstacles and foster dialogue between the 'persona' and the 'anima', recognizing the distinct essence of each beyond superficial aspects. In the group and interpersonal relationships, this dialogue corresponds to accepting the continual and profound changes that follow the evolution of the individuation process.

Protagonist   The narrator and actor of one or more scenes that are enacted in psychodrama is known as the protagonist. Usually the **conductor** selects the protagonist or protagonists to work on in the individual sessions. The choice is instinctive but based on the sociometry of the group itself. The protagonist chosen is the one whose themes seem to best catalyse the group's energy and attention, effecting the most resonance. The sociometric choice can be made more or less explicitly through questions or play. However, the conductor's choice is based on what he or she seems to be picking up on from the group – the attitudes, mimicked expressions, postures, associations or other less explicit messages that appear to indicate the themes that have more widespread emotional impact at that time. As a response to analogous messages after the first scene, the conductor may propose one or more successive scenes to the protagonist that would go deeper into the problem, or may work on other participants for whom the enacted scene has evoked memories or images that helped bring forth a greater emotional intensity. This does not mean that the protagonist who opened the session has been forgotten but simply that he or she is allowed to let the contents that have emerged settle along with the emotions, images, memories, and feelings evoked by the scene in the expectation that they can reach a clearer formulation. This wait can help the initial protagonist gather eventual responses to be given back as the theme develops later. Substantially, *the attention focused on the protagonist is always constantly balanced by an attention towards the group as a whole*. Likewise, the themes played on **stage** by individual participants are the themes of the protagonist that simultaneously reflect those of the group as a whole. The images that emerge and the scenes that are enacted represent in themselves a kind of response that is always an opening towards other questions and towards the problems or conflict that the first protagonist introduced. The theme will be returned to him or her enhanced by the new resonance and the faceting revealed by the group and opened towards new creative potential to formulate new hypotheses.

Psychodramatic scene and play   Various scenes are put on through play and follow each other during the course of a 90-minute psychodrama session. The scenes consist in performing some relatively short pieces from lives that have been lived as well as memories, dreams, and dialogues with oneself or with others. For the most part, the scenes that are played are proposed by the **protagonist** who has introduced the theme or the problem that he or she is interested in working on. At times, however, the **conductor** may invite the protagonist to focus on something that may have merely seemed tangential and so cause the protagonist to play a scene different from the one originally embarked on – sometimes involving a detail or something that was mentioned as an association. For example, participants can pass from a dream to the playing of a scene from real life or vice versa. This occurs mainly when the conductor feels the need to overcome rationalizing defences. The content of the scene that is played can involve differing time frames: a recent recollection, an impression or fantasy that has to do with the 'here and now', a memory that dates back to several months or many years ago, or a sequence from a dream that belongs to the timeless space of the world of dreams. It often happens that a scene from a dream may be followed by a scene from a protagonist's real-life experiences that the dream seems to evoke. It may even happen that the following scenes relate to dreams or memories evoked in other participants that seem to develop the same theme. Sometimes the scenes – both those involving dreams and those from real life – may appear to be evoked by the very reality of the group as a whole and its history, which continually intertwines with the history and reality of the individual participants. Playing scenes causes the dreams or memories that belong to the dreamers' inner worlds to become concrete realities for the group to share. For this reason, analytical work can be directed along parallel lines towards the protagonist, the group as a whole, and the individual participants and can focus on the inner- or outer-world aspects in the individual group members. The actors are 'the protagonist' – the narrator of what the scene is about – and the **'auxiliary egos'** chosen by the protagonist from among the participants to play the various parts, defined as **'roles'**. During the dramatic playing of the scenes the conductor focuses on the emotional states and subsequent transformations that seem most significant in order to gather in the most profound and complex aspects of what has been narrated. Over the course of the play the protagonist is invited to make successive 'role exchanges' with one or more characters that are participating in the scene itself, thus giving him or her the chance to experience personally the emotional states and perspectives of even his or her antagonists and to gather new nuances from them. After the play, the actor-participants recount their feedback – the moods, feelings, and emotions that they experienced in the roles that they played.

Role The role is the part that the **protagonist** of the scene to be played assigns to some of the other group participants. A scene is chosen and then constructed. Here the characters, the feelings in the air, the objects, and the atmosphere take shape bit by bit on the psychodramatic **stage** as the setting is described and structured. The participants thus function as **'auxiliary egos'**, interpreting the various roles – i.e. the parts that the protagonist assigns. Aside from human characters, some participants may be called on to play the roles of inanimate objects in order to explore the symbolic and emotional significance that these can have for the protagonist. Emotions, feelings, or somatic symptoms can be represented for the same reason.

Self The Self represents the ultimate aim of the process of **individuation** in as far as it is the realization of the totality innate in each person. The Self is the symbol of completeness and unity. As such it is the union of the conscious and the unconscious and the synthesis of all opposites. It is therefore something indescribable and connected with the idea of the sacred. It is expressed through symbols – the mandala, the circle, fire, etc. – that have the feature of **numinosity**, which means they have the ability to attract the contents of the consciousness totally by developing, if only for brief moments, an ecstatic contemplation, as might occur in some vision-like experiences and strongly emotion-packed dreams. Images of the Self include the representations of divinities in every epoch and culture and, simultaneously, the manifestations of the sacred inside each individual.

Shadow   In Jungian terms the shadow is what stands in antithesis to everything that is put out into the light in order to adapt socially to the values of the collective consciousness. In the form of an 'autonomous **complex**' the shadow gathers to itself everything that has been removed from the consciousness of the ego and 'sacrificed to adaptation'. It contains traits and behaviour patterns that the conscious ego attempts to repress or ignore. As an **archetypal image**, the shadow is at the same level as the **anima**. It is relatively autonomous in relation to the conscious ego, which it stands up against. Thus the shadow appears to be also granted a life of its own in its interactions. The shadow is a receptacle for everything that is discarded because it disturbs and clashes with conscious values. For this reason, the shadow often is a carrier of a strong charge of energy and of very positive resources. The shadow frequently appears in dreams in the shapes of characters that are attributed with rough, primitive, strongly instinctual, vulgar, and degrading characteristics. The shadow often takes on markedly caricature-like features. The repugnance and disgust that these dream characters arouse is linked to the fact that they display the same features that the dreamers refuse to accept in themselves. Analytic work tends to free the energy that this repression has imprisoned by allowing the dialogue between the conscious and the unconscious to flow. When people reclaim their own shadows, they take a fundamental step on their individuative paths. In psychodrama the shadow is often unmasked through the projections of the other participants on to the group, through the invitation to play undesired **roles**, and through the enactment of scenes or dreams that imply role exchange.

Sharing   Sharing usually follows the dramatization of every scene. However, a **conductor** may sometimes choose to pass on to another scene quickly when he or she thinks this would be more likely to exploit the emotional energy that has just been mobilized while it is still 'hot'. In this case, the conductor would take up the sharing later. Essentially, sharing goes in two directions. The first has to do with the emotions, sentiments, and feelings experienced in the scenes in relation to the **roles** that were assigned in the play and in the eventual role exchanges. At this stage it is important, as much as possible, that the **protagonists** work as '**auxiliary egos**' and thus are able to give back what they imagine is 'faithful' to the script assigned them while avoiding personal interference and projections. This is done in order to give the protagonists the feedback that would allow them more deeply to grasp the meaning of the relationship that was played in the scene. This may happen whether the scene was related to real people who take part in their lives, to dream images, or to something else that was represented in the scene. The other direction of the sharing usually, but not always, follows the first. In contrast, this enters the real situation of the individual group members as such: that is to say, it is more related to their own personal features. It therefore can pertain to feelings and emotions experienced that seem to each of the participants to be more related to themselves than to the protagonist. It can also pertain to personal associations that may or may not be the topics of successive scenes. Usually sharing does not involve all the potential feedback in reaction to the scenes played in a session. Here too the conductor has to choose to make more room for those instances of feedback that seem to be most meaningful, most 'emotionally charged' and most pertinent to the theme of the session and to the problems that the protagonist brought in. It is usually the protagonists themselves who choose either to speak first or to hear the group's feedback first at the end of the dramatization of a scene. At the end of every session it is customary to leave some space for feelings or emotions that some participants might feel are still up in the air – those that are strictly personal and those that come as the feedback of an auxiliary ego. Other feelings that may be less immediate return, instead, more frequently in successive sessions in the form of thoughts, reflections or dreams.

Stage   The stage where the dramatic action takes place is the physical space delineated by the participants sitting in a circle. In this position they all are equidistant from the centre where the scenes take place. At the same time they all can see the others' faces and likewise be seen. The circle has a kind of 'magic' capacity to involve people. Each participant knows that he or she is part of the group and so is particularly important for it. Thus the space assumes the aspects of a 'temenos' – i.e. a kind of sacred reserve where the scenes represent the celebration of a kind of ritual performed for its participants. On stage there are some elements that remain fixed – the timed recurrence of the sessions, their constant duration, and the physical space that borders them. All this contributes to create a kind of frame and ritual-like quality. In this way, in this scenic space transformed into a kind of steady 'temenos', the element of change is represented by the scenes that are enacted. These are in a continuous development that narrates and reflects the group's history through the participants' experiences and dreams. Images from the participants' lives and fantasies find room for themselves on stage, where they are joined by images coming out of the unconscious as dream images and then incarnated in the concrete reality of the **psychodramatic play**. Thus the stage functions as the meeting place of the concrete reality represented, on the one hand, by the group as a whole that marks its borders and by its individual participants and, on the other hand, by the reality of the inner world of the **protagonists**. Their unconscious images in their subjective reality are expressed through scenic representation. In as much as the stage is a symbolic space representing the 'heart' or centre of the group's space where its energy gathers and increases, it sometimes appears in the participants' dreams transfigured by the emotions that have been projected on to it.

Unconscious, collective   By collective unconscious is meant the deepest level of the unconscious. It represents a kind of heritage shared by all humanity. Its root is represented by **archetypes** – archaic psychic structures that appear through the flourishing of highly emotionally charged symbolic images. Archetypes express themselves through myths, dreams, and fables. Archetypal images often emerge during the enactment of dreams in psychodrama scenes. When this happens, intense emotions may move the group.

Unconscious, personal   Jungian thought distinguishes the personal unconscious from the **collective unconscious**. By personal unconscious is meant the gathering of psychic contents that have been repressed, that have never crossed the threshold of consciousness, and that have limited themselves to subliminal perceptions. This is a concept that shows significant affinity with the Freudian unconscious. In regard to this, what Jung defines as 'autonomous **complexes**' establish themselves. These are linked to an individual's more personal problems. The contents of the personal unconscious emerge easily in psychodrama through the enactment of scenes.

Uroboros   The mythical figure of a serpent or dragon that eats its own tail is called a urobos. It can be used as a symbol of **individuation**, understood as a circular process closed in itself that follows the evolution of the consciousness from primordial chaos along parallel lines. The end of the individuation process is death, understood in a positive sense as the passage into a state analogous with birth or as the closure of the circle through the annihilation of the individual consciousness in the uroboric one–everything that represents the primordial entity. In group analysis the uroboros represents the most regressive maternal aspects. These are affective and welcoming, but can also be the enveloping, suffocating, and non-differentiating aspects projected on to the group itself. The uroboric circle is a mandalic symbol that contains opposites; while it allows people to face up to the wounds that come out of conflicts, it is also the carrier of dependence and limits.

Warming up   A cluster of techniques that aim to facilitate communication among group participants. Warming up is rarely employed in continuous psychodrama groups, but can sometimes be used when situations seem to be stalled. As in individual analysis, it is more often preferable to face silences, even long ones, in which contents take shape in the participants' minds. These may be harder and sometimes more painful to take on, but also more significant. Facing moments of emptiness and expectation in the group can therefore cause deeper themes to emerge. However, the warming up technique can be used frequently, although not obligatorily, in workshops where the participants hardly know each other, in situations where the group is not homogenous and its participants need to be better integrated, or in situations where the group participants are not at all used to working with psychodramatic techniques and so need a more gentle first impact and start-up. Warming up thus allows the participants to relate to each other a little by coming closer to each other progressively.

Bibliography

Ancelin Schützenberger, Anne (1970). *Précis de Psychodrame* [Outline of Psychodrama]. Paris: Editions Universitaires.

—— (1972). *Lo psicodramma*. Florence: Martinelli. (Italian translation of Ancelin 1970)

—— (1975). *Introduction au Jeu du rôle* [Introduction to Role-playing]. Toulouse: Eduard Privat.

—— (1978a). *Il corpo e il gruppo* [The Body and the Group]. Rome: Astrolabio.

Ancona, Leonardo (1983). 'I fondamenti della gruppoanalisi' [The fundamentals of group analysis], in Franco Di Maria and Giralomo Loverso (eds) *Il piccolo gruppo* [The Small Group]. Rome: Bulzoni.

Bachelard, Gaston (1948a). *La terre et les Rêveries de la Repos* [The Earth and the Dreams of Rest]. Paris: José Corti.

—— (1948b). *La terre et les Rêveries de la Volonté* [The Earth and the Dreams of the Will]. Paris: José Corti.

—— (1964). *The Psychoanalysis of Fire*. Boston: Beacon.

—— (1987). *L'Eau et les Rêves*. Paris: J. Corti.

—— (1988a). *Fragments d'une poétique du feu* [Fragments of a Poetics of Fire]. Paris: PUF.

—— (1988b). *Air and Dreams: An Essay on the Imagination of Movement*. Dallas: Dallas Institute Publications.

—— (1994). *Water and Dreams*. Dallas: Dallas Institute Publications. (Translation of Bachelard 1987)

Barz, Elynor (1988). *Selbstbegegnung im Spiel* [The Encounter with the Self in Play]. Zurich: Kreuz.

Bateson, Gregory (1972). *Steps to an Ecology of the Mind*. San Francisco: Chandler.

Baudouin, Charles (1963). *L'oeuvre de Jung et la psychologie complexe* [The Work of Jung and Complex Psychology]. Paris: Payot.

Benedetto, Nadia (ed.) (1994). *Pensare l'apprendere: La formazione in gruppoanalisi* [Thinking Learning: Training in Group Analysis]. Turin: Upsel.

Bernard, Ernst (1978). *Mitobiografia* [Myth-biography]. Milan: Adelphi.

Bettelheim, Bruno (1976). *The Uses of Enchantment: The Meaning and Importance of Fairy Tales*. New York: Knopf.

Bion, Wilfred R. (1971). *Experiences in Group and Other Papers*. London: Tavistock.

Boria, G. (1983). *Tele: Manuale di psicodramma classica* [Tele: Manual of Classic Psychodrama]. Milan: France Angeli.

—— (1991). *Spontaneità e incontro nella vita e negli scritti di J.L. Moreno* [Spontaneity and Encounter in the Life and Writings of J.P. Moreno]. Padua: Upsel.

Bustos, Dalmiro (1981). *Signification del encuentro en Psicoterapia Psicodramatica* [The Meaning of the Encounter in Psychodramatic Psychotherapy]. La Plata: Instituto Psicodrama Buenos Aires-La Plata.

—— (1985). *Nuevos Rumbos en Psicoterapia Psicodramatica* [New Roads in Psychodramatic Psychotherapy]. La Plata: Momento.

Cook, Roger (1974). *The Tree of Life: Symbol of the Centre.* London. Thames and Hudson.

Croce, E.B. (1900). *Il volo della farfalla* [The Flight of the Butterfly]. Rome: Borla.

Deacon, A.B. (1934). 'Geometrical drawings from Malekula and other islands of the New Hebrides', *Journal of the Anthropological Institute*, 64.

De Marè, P.B. (1994). *Prospettive di psicoterapia di gruppo* [Views on Group Psychotherapy]. Rome: Astrolabio.

Di Maria, Franco and Lavanco, G. (1994). *Nel nome del gruppo* [In the Name of the Group]. Milan: Franco Angeli.

Di Salvo, S. (1995). *Iniziazione sciamanica, initiazioine analitica* [Shamanic initiation, analytic initiation]. Turin: Cortina.

Eliade, Mircea (1942). *Mitul Reintegrării* [The Myth of Reintegration]. Bucharest: Vremea.

—— (1963). *Patterns in Comparative Religion.* New York: New American Library-Meridian.

—— (1965). *Rites and Symbols of Initiation: The Mysteries of Birth and Rebirth.* New York: Harper Torchbooks.

—— (1967). *Myths, Dreams, and Mysteries.* New York: Harper Torchbooks.

—— (1969). *The Two and the One.* New York: Harper Torchbooks.

—— (1974). *Shamanism: Archaic Techniques of Ecstasy.* Princeton: Princeton University Press.

—— (1978). *A History of Religious Ideas. Vol. 1: From the Stone Age to the Eleusinian Mysteries.* Chicago: University of Chicago Press.

—— (1987). *The Sacred and the Profane: The Nature of Religion.* New York: Harper & Row.

—— (1989). *Il mito della reintegrazione* [The Myth of Reintegration]. Milan: Jaka. (Translation of Eliade 1942).

—— (1991). *The Myth of the Eternal Return or, Cosmos and History.* Princeton: Princeton University Press.

Espina Barrio, J.A. (1995). *Nacimiento y Desarollo* [Birth and Development]. Salamanca: Amarù.

Foulkes, Siegmund Heinz (1965). *Therapeutic Group Analysis.* New York: International Universities Press.

—— (1975). *Group-analytic Psychotherapy: Methods and Principles.* New York: Gordon and Breach.

Franz, Marie-Louise von (1972). *Problems of Feminine Psychology in Fairy Tales.* New York: Spring.

—— (1983). *Das Weibliche im Märchen.* Stuttgart. (German original of Franz 1972)

—— (1990). *Individuation in Fairy Tales.* Boston: Shambala.

—— (1996). *The Interpretation of Fairy Tales.* Boston: Shambala.

Frazer, James G. (1922). *The Golden Bough: A Study in Magic and Religion.* Abridged edn (2 vols). New York: Macmillan.

Freud, Sigmund (1994). *The Interpretation of Dreams.* New York: Modern Library.

Gasca, Giulio and Gasseau, Maurizio (1991). *Lo Psicodramma jungiano* [Jungian Psychodrama]. Turin: Bollati Boringhieri.

Gasca, Giulio, Gasseau, Maurizio and Scategni, Wilma (1988). 'Lo pscicodramma individuativo' [Individuative psychodrama], *Psichiatria generale dell'età evolutiva*, 26.

Gifford, Douglas (1983). *Warriors, Gods, and Spirits from Central and South American Mythology*. London: Peter Lowe-Eurobook.

Gocci, Giovanni (1989). *Gruppi di individuazione* [Individuation Groups]. Florence: Il Ventaglio.

Goethe, Johann Wolfgang von (1951). *Conversations of Goethe with Eckermann*. New York: Dutton.

Gonda, Jan (1960). *Die Religionen Indiens. 1. Veda und älterer Hinduismus* [The Religions of India: The Veda and early Hinduism]. Stuttgart: Verlag W. Kohlhammer.

The Grimms' German Folk Tales (1969). (Francis P. Magoun and Alexander Krappe, trans.). Carbondale: Southern Illinois University Press.

Heraclitus of Ephesus (1969). *The Fragments of the Work of Heraclitus of Ephesus: On Nature . . . and By Water*. Chicago: Argonaut.

Hesse, Hermann (1963). *Steppenwolf*. New York: Modern Library. [Original edn 1927.]

Hillman, James. (1979). *The Dream and the Underworld*. New York: Harper & Row.

—— (1992). 'Healing fiction', in R.P. Sugg (ed.) *Jungian Literary Criticism*. Evanston: Northwestern University Press.

Holmes, P. and Karp, M. (1991). *Psychodrama: Inspiration and Technique*. London: Routledge.

—— (1994). *Psychodrama Since Moreno*. London: Routledge.

Janet, Pierre (1925). *Études experimentales. 1. Névroses et idées fixes* [Experimental Studies. 1. Neuroses and Fixed Ideas], 4th edn. Paris: Alcan. [Original edn 1904–08.]

Jung, Carl Gustav (1967–78). *The Collected Works of C.G. Jung* (Vols 1–20). Princeton: Princeton University Press.

—— Vol. 5. *Symbols of Transformation*.

—— Vol. 7. *Two Essays of Analytical Psychology*.

—— Vol. 8. *The Structure and Dynamics of the Psyche*.

—— Vol. 9. Part 1. *The Archetypes and the Collective Unconscious*.

—— Vol. 9. Part 2. *Aion, Researches into the Phenomenology of the Self*.

—— Vol. 11. *Psychology and Religion, West and East*.

—— Vol. 14. *Mysterium Coniunctionis, an Inquiry into the Separation and Synthesis of Psychic Opposites in Alchemy*.

—— Vol. 16. *The Practice of Psychotherapy*.

—— (1975). *Letters. Vol. 2: 1951–1961*. Princeton: Princeton University Press.

Kellermann, Peter Felix (1992). *Focus on Psychodrama: The Therapeutic Aspects of Psychodrama*. London: Jessica Kingsley.

Kerényi, Karoly (1949). 'Mensch und Maske' [People and masks]. *Eranos Jahrbuch 1948*, Vol. 16. Zurich: Rhein.

Kipper, D.A. (1986). *Psychotherapy through Clinical Role Playing*. New York: Brunner/Mazel.

Lauf, Detlef Ingo (1976). *Tibetan Sacred Art*. Berkeley: Shambala.

—— (1992). *Il libro tibetano dei morti*. Rome: Mediterranee. (Translation of Lauf 1976).

Lebovici, S. (1980). *Terapia psicoanalitica di gruppo* [Group Psychoanalytic Therapy]. Milan: Feltrinelli.

Leeuw, Gerardus van der (1938). *Religion in Essence and Manifestation*. London: Allen and Unwin.

Lemoine, P. and Lemoine, G. (1973). *Le Psychodrame* [Psychodrama]. Paris: Laffont.

Leutz, Grete (1985). *Mettre sa Vie en scène* [Putting One's Life on the Stage]. Paris: EPI.

—— (1986). *Psychodrama: Theorie und Praxis* [Psychodrama: Theory and Practice]. Berlin: Springer.

Lévy-Bruhl, Lucien (1938). *L'Expérience mystique et les symboles chez les primitifs*. Paris: n.p.

—— (1966). *The 'Soul' of the Primitive*. Chicago: Henry Regnery. (Translation of Lévy-Bruhl 1938.)

Lo Verso, Giralomo (1984). *Il gruppo, una prospettiva dinamica e clinica* [The Group: A Dynamic and Clinical Perspective]. Milan: Giuffrè.

Marineau, Renè (1989). *Jacob Levi Moreno 1889–1974: Father of Psychodrama, Sociometry and Group Psychotherapy*. London: Tavistock-Routledge.

Mauss, Marcel (n.d.). *A General Theory of Magic*. New York: W.W. Norton. (Translation of Mauss and Hubert 1909)

Mauss, M. and Hubert, Henri (1909). 'La représentation du temps dans la religion et la magie' [The representation of time in religion and magic], in *Mélanges d'histoire des religions* [Various Essays on the History of Religion]. Paris: n.p.

Menarini, R., Ancona, L. and Pontaldi, C. (1992). *La costruzione del Sé dal vertice dei campi mentali familiari–gruppali–terapeutici. Le matrici relazionali del Sé* [The Construction of the Self at the Summit of Family–Group–Therapeutic Mental Fields: The Relational Matrixes of the Self]. Rome: Il pensiero scientifico.

Menegazzo, Carlos Maria (1976). *El desarrollo dramatico del proceso de identidad. El modelo evolutivo dramatico de Moreno* [Dramatic Development of the Process of Identity: Moreno's Dramatic-evolutionary Model]. Buenos Aires: Instituto A.A. Meneghino.

—— (1991). *Umbrales de plenitud* [Thresholds of Plenty]. Buenos Aires: Fundacion Vinculo.

Montesarchio, G. and Sardi, P. (1987). *Dal teatro della spontaneità allo psicodramma classico* [From the Theatre of Spontaneity to Classical Psychodrama]. Milan: Angeli.

Moreno, Jacob Levi (1946). *Psychodrama*. Vol 1. Beacon, NY: Beacon House.

—— (1947). *The Theater of Spontaneity: An Introduction to Psychodrama*. Beacon, NY: Beacon House.

—— (1951). *Sociometry: Experimental Method and the Science of Society*. Beacon, NY: Beacon House.

Moreno, Jacob Levi and Moreno, Zerka Toeman (1959). *Psychodrama*. Vol. 2. Beacon, NY: Beacon House.

—— (1969). *Psychodrama*. Vol. 3. Beacon, NY: Beacon House.

Moreno, Zerka (1978). 'Psychodrama', in H. Mullan and M. Rosenbaum (eds) *Group Psychotherapy: Theory and Practice*. New York: Free Press.

Moretta, Angelo (1982). *Miti indiani* [Indian Myths]. Milan: Longanesi.

Napolitani, Diego (1987). *Individualità e gruppalità* [Individuality and Group-ness]. Turin: Bollati Boringhieri.

Neumann, Erich (1955). *The Great Mother: An Analysis of the Archetype*. Princeton: Princeton University Press.

—— (1993). *The Origins and History of Consciousness*. Princeton: Princeton University Press. (Original edition 1949).

Pauletta D'Anna, Gian Mario (1990). *Modelli psicoanalitici del gruppo* [Psychoanalytic Models of the Group]. Milan: Guerini e Associati.

Pines, Malcolm (1983). *The Evolution of Group Analysis*. Boston: Routledge.

Pines, Malcolm and Rafaelson, Lise (eds) (1982). *The Individual and the Group: Boundaries and Interrelations*. New York: Plenum.

Propp, Vladimir (1946). *Istoriceskie korni volsebnoj skazki* [Historical Roots of the Wondertale]. Leningrad: Leningradskij gosudarstvennyi universitet.

—— (1984). 'Historical roots of the wondertale: Premises and the wondertale as a whole', in Anatoly Liberman (ed.) *Theory and History of Folklore*. Minneapolis: University of Minnesota Press. (Translation of Propp 1946, chapters 1 & 10.)

—— (1985). *Le radici storiche dei racconti di fate*. Turin: Boringhieri. (Translation of Propp 1946.)

Raine, Kathleen (1958). *William Blake*. London: Longmans, Green.

Quaglino, G.P., Casagrande, S. and Castellano, A. (1992). *Gruppo di lavoro, lavoro di gruppo* [Work Group, Group Work]. Milan: Cortina.

Ripellino, A.M. (1981). 'L'omino delle acque' [The Little Man of the Waters], in Frantisek Langer (ed.) *Leggende praghesi* [Legends of Prague]. Rome: e/o.

Rojas Bermudez, Jaime (1979). 'Introducción al nucleo del yo' [Introduction to the nucleus of the ego], *Cuadernos de Psicoterapia* [Buenos Aires], 9 (1–2).

Romano, A. (1975). *Studi sull'ombra* [Studies on the Shadow]. Venice: Marsilio.

Rosati, Ottavio (1985). 'J.L. Moreno e gli action methods' [J.L. Moreno and action methods], in J.L. Moreno *Manuale di Psicodramma* [Psychodrama, vol. 1]. Rome: Astrolabio.

Thompson, Stith (1946). *The Folktale*. New York: Holt, Reinhart & Winston.

Traveni, Anna Maria and Benedetto, Nadia (eds) (1986). *Gruppi e Psicosi.* [Groups and Psychoses]. Turin: Ar. Form. Usl 1–23.

Warner, Elizabeth (1995). *Heroes, Monsters and Other Worlds from Russian Mythology*. London: Peter Lowe-Eurobook.

Winnicott, Donald Woods (1971). *Playing and Reality*. London: Tavistock.

Wundt, Willhelm (1916). *Elements of Folk Psychology*. New York: Macmillan.

Yablonsky, L. (1976). *Psychodrama: Resolving Emotional Problems Through Role Playing*. New York: Basic Books.

Yalom, I.D. (1975). *The Theory and Practice of Group Psychotherapy*, 2nd edn New York: Basic Books.

Zoja, Luigi (1985). *Nascere non basta* [Being Born is not Enough]. Milan: Raffaello Cartina.

Name Index

Aesculapius 89
Ancelin Schützenberger, A. 13, 15
Apuleius 9
Aristotle 15
Artemidorus 101
Artusi, P. 76

Bachelard, G. 105, 111–12, 114, 116, 126,
    129–32, 143
Barz. E. 14
Baudouin, C. 16
Bergson, H. 16
Bernard, E. 79
Blake, W. 120

Castenda, C. 120
Clement of Alexandria 9
Cook, R. 59, 101

Deacon, A.B. 96

Eliade, M. 1, 7–8, 25–30, 38–9, 41–4, 57,
    65–7, 69–70, 74, 81, 87, 94–7, 99–101,
    104, 110, 116, 119–20, 123–4, 127,
    131, 138, 140

Franz, M.L. von 22, 54–5, 98, 129
Frazer, J.G. 7, 8, 9
Freud, S. 12–13, 23, 103, 142

Gasca, G. 14, 20–1, 142
Gasseau, M. 14, 21, 142
Gifford, D. 59
Goethe, J.W. Von 109
Gonda, J. 132

Heraclitus 100, 115
Herodotus 7

Hesiod 100
Hesse, H. 22, 93
Hillman, J. 10, 23–4, 29, 39, 41, 44, 47,
    77–9, 90, 98, 100–01, 103, 111–12,
    114–15, 142
Hippolytus 9

Illing, H. 14

Janet, P. 117
Jung, C.G. 14, 16, 19, 22, 37, 74;
    CW5 40–1, 129; CW7 81;
    CW8 15, 17–18, 21–2, 141;
    CW9 38; CW11 116; CW14 62;
    CW16 62, 115

Kerényi, K. 8–10, 75

Lactantius 8
Lauf, I. 116
Layard, J.W. 96
Lebovci, C. 13
Lévy-Bruhl, L. 27

Mauss, M. 41–2
Moreno, J. 10–19, 125
Moretta, A. 129

Neumann, E. 39–40, 43–4, 53–4, 62, 67,
    84–6, 120, 134, 138

Plato 44
Plutarch 70
Propp, V. 54–5, 79–80, 101–2

Raine, K. 120
Ripellino, A.M. 117
Romano, A. 70, 142

Subject Index

Dream Index